THE NEW BIBLE
C URE
WEIGHT LOSS

DON COLBERT, MD

SILOAM

Most CHARISMA HOUSE BOOK GROUP products are available at special quantity discounts for bulk purchase for sales promotions, premiums, fund-raising, and educational needs. For details, write Charisma House Book Group, 600 Rinehart Road, Lake Mary, Florida 32746, or telephone (407) 333-0600.

THE NEW BIBLE CURE FOR WEIGHT LOSS by Don Colbert, MD
Published by Siloam
Charisma Media/Charisma House Book Group
600 Rinehart Road, Lake Mary, Florida 32746
www.charismahouse.com

Library of Congress Cataloging-in-Publication Data
Colbert, Don.
  The new Bible cure for weight loss / Don Colbert, MD.
      pages cm
  Includes bibliographical references and index.
  ISBN 978-1-61638-616-0 (trade paper) -- ISBN 978-1-62136-529-7 (e-book)
  1. Weight loss--Popular works. 2. Weight loss--Alternative treatment--Popular works. 3. Weight loss--Religious aspects--Christianity. I. Title. II. Title: Weight loss.
  RM222.2.C5522 2013
  613.2'5--dc23
                                                            2013013911

16 17 18 19 20 — 10 9 8 7 6 5 4
Printed in the United States of America

CONTENTS

YOU ARE GOD'S MASTERPIECE!

BEFORE THE FINGER of God touched the oceans with unimaginable creative power, God envisioned you in His heart. He saw you and all you could be one day through the power of His supernatural grace.

You are God's masterpiece, designed according to an eternal plan so awesome that it's beyond your ability to comprehend. Have you ever wondered what He saw in His mind when He created you? What was the perfection of purpose and plan He intended?

Now close your eyes and see yourself. For one moment you have no bondages, no imperfections, no shortcomings. Your body is as lean and healthy as it could possibly be. What do you look like? Is that the person God had in mind?

If you've struggled with obesity all of your life, you may not even be able to imagine yourself free of the bondage of unwanted fat. But God can. Don't you think that if God is powerful enough to create you and the entire universe that you see around you, He is also able to help you overcome all of your personal bondages? Of course He is!

That's what this Bible Cure is all about. It is a plan of godly principles, wisdom, and scriptural advice to help deliver you from an unhealthy lifestyle and future ill health and to give you the freedom and joy of a healthy, fit, more attractive you!

AN OBESITY EPIDEMIC

If you have a weight problem, you're not alone. The terms *over-weight* and *obese* are defined using the body mass index (BMI), which evaluates a person's weight relative to height. Various health organizations, including the Centers for Disease Control and Prevention (CDC) and the National Institutes of Health (NIH), define an overweight adult as having a BMI between 25 and 29.9, while an obese adult is anyone with a BMI of 30 or higher.[1]

In the last several years America has experienced an alarming arise in obesity. Two-thirds of American adults are overweight or obese, and 30 percent of children age eleven or younger are overweight.[2] This should concern everyone, particularly those of us who professes Jesus as Savior and Lord. God revealed His divine will for each of us through the apostle John, who wrote, "Beloved, I pray that you may prosper in all things and be in health, just as your soul prospers" (3 John 2). With obesity at almost epidemic proportions, surely we are missing God's best.

A DEADLY KILLER

Research tells us that, in the United States, an estimated 300,000 deaths per year are attributed to obesity.[3] Obesity also comes with a fat price tag (pun intended). People considered obese pay $1,429 more (42 percent) in health care costs than normal weight individuals.[4] And as shocking as all this sounds, no dollar amount can do justice to the real damage being done. Being overweight or obese increases your risk of developing thirty-five major diseases, particularly type 2 diabetes, heart disease, stroke, arthritis, hypertension, acid reflux, sleep apnea,

Alzheimer's, infertility, erectile dysfunction, and gallbladder disease—plus more than a dozen forms of cancer.

Besides obesity's physical implications, it carries a social and psychological impact. Obese individuals generally contend with more rejection and prejudice. Often they are overlooked for promotions or not even hired because of physical appearance. Most obese people struggle daily with issues of self-worth and self-image. They feel unattractive and unappreciated and are at an increased risk of depression. Many of us have watched the humiliation an obese person experiences trying to squeeze into an airplane, stadium, or automobile seat that is too small. Maybe you have been that person. If so, you know how obesity can affect the way others treat you and how you treat yourself.

POWER FOR SUCCESS

Instead of looking for the next new-and-improved medication to manage obesity-related disease, we need to get to the root of the problem, which is our diet, lifestyle, and waistline. The standard American diet is full of empty carbohydrates, sugars, fats, excessive proteins, and calories, and it is low in nutrient content. Combined with our poor diet is a lack of physical activity and excessive stress that usually raises cortisol levels. Because of this increase of cortisol, many are developing toxic belly fat, which increases their risk for incurring a host of other diseases, including diabetes.

This simple Bible Cure provides all you need for health and successful weight loss to help you become the person you saw or imagined when you closed your eyes. With fresh understanding, proper nutrition, exercise, and supplements you can find all the physical elements you need for radical change. Mixed together with the power of God found in prayer and Scripture, you will discover strength for success that is beyond your own ability.

Originally published as *The Bible Cure for Weight Loss and Muscle Gain* in 2000, *The New Bible Cure for Weight Loss* has been revised and updated with the latest medical research on ways to reduce your waistline, control your weight, and rid yourself of the toxic body fat that leads to so many diseases. If you compare it side by side with the previous edition, you'll see that it's also larger, allowing me to expand greatly upon the information provided in the previous edition and provide you with a deeper understanding of what you face and how to overcome it.

Unchanged from the previous edition are the timeless, life-changing, and healing scriptures throughout this book that will strengthen and encourage your spirit and soul. The proven principles, truths, and guidelines in these passages anchor the practical and medical insights also contained in this book. They will effectively focus your prayers, thoughts, and actions so you can step into God's plan of divine health for you—a plan that includes victory over obesity.

Another change since the original *The Bible Cure for Weight Loss and Muscle Gain* was published is that I've released two important books on weight loss, *The Rapid Waist Reduction Diet* and *Dr. Colbert's "I Can Do This" Diet*. I encourage you to read those books, because they delve even deeper into the changes that will empower you to lose weight and keep it off. I also recommend my book *The Seven Pillars of Health* because the principles it contains are the foundation to healthy living that will affect all areas of your life. It sets the stage for everything you will ever read in any other book I've published—including this one.

I pray that these spiritual and practical suggestions for health, nutrition, and fitness will bring wholeness to your life, increase your spiritual understanding, and strengthen your ability to worship and serve God.

There is much you can do to change the course of your health. As you learn about obesity, understand its causes, and take the practical, positive steps detailed in this book, you will defeat obesity in your life and discover the abundant life promised by Jesus when He said, "I have come that they may have life, and that they may have it more abundantly" (John 10:10).

Now is the time to run to the battle with fresh confidence, renewed determination, and the wonderful knowledge that God is real, alive, and more powerful than any sickness or disease. It is my prayer that my suggestions and guidelines will help improve your health, nutritional habits, and fitness practices. This combination will bring wholeness to your life. I pray that they will deepen your fellowship with God and strengthen your ability to worship and serve Him.

—Don Colbert, MD

A **BIBLE CURE** Prayer for You

I pray that God will fill you with hope, encouragement, and wisdom as you read this book. May He give you the willpower to make healthy choices about your nutrition, exercise, and lifestyle. May He strengthen your resolve to maintain a healthy weight and not to overtax your body with excessive weight. I pray that you live a long and prosperous life living in divine health so that you may fulfill your purpose and serve the Lord. Amen.

Chapter 1

DID YOU KNOW?—
UNDERSTANDING OBESITY

T HE BIBLE INSTRUCTS us to be wise in our eating habits: "Whether you eat or drink, or whatever you do, do all to the glory of God" (1 Cor. 10:31). The way you eat, drink, and care for the body that God gave you can bring glory to Him for this wonderful gift.

Chances are that if you are struggling with obesity, you may have been waging a war with it all of your life. By now you realize that you need more than a good dieting program. You need power to enforce it. You need the strength it takes to change a lifetime of poor eating habits and the discipline to stay with it. This Bible Cure pathway to wholeness not only provides the information necessary for a healthier, trimmer body, but it also provides insight into an endless source of power to insure success. Stop limiting yourself to your own strength. The Bible reveals a better way:

> I can do all things through Christ who strengthens me.
>
> —PHILIPPIANS 4:13

Gaining new power in your battle against obesity must begin with gaining fresh understanding of the causes for obesity.

WHY WE EAT TOO MUCH

Being overweight has many causes. Some are biological. You might be predisposed to obesity through genetics and body metabolism. Some of the causes are psychological.

Emotional eating

You also may be emotionally dependent on food for comfort during times of stress, crisis, anxiety, loneliness, and a host of other emotions. If overeating has an emotional component in your life, you probably grew up hearing statements such asthe following:

- "Eat something; it will make you feel better."
- "Clean your plate, or you can't leave the table."
- "If you're good, you will get dessert."
- "If you don't eat everything, you will be impolite to the host or hostess."
- "If you stop crying, I'll give you ice cream."

> Through the LORD's mercies we are not consumed, because His compassions fail not. They are new every morning; great is Your faithfulness.
> —LAMENTATIONS 3:22–23

The list of unhealthy childhood motivations can be endless. But whether the causes of your weight problem are genetic or psychological, you are not bound to your past. Today is a new day, filled with fresh hope for an entirely new way of thinking and living. Begin considering what lifestyle factors might be contributing to your situation.

A sedentary lifestyle

Another cause of obesity is the increasingly sedentary lifestyle in our society. In an agricultural or industrial culture hard work gives people plenty of exercise during the day. In our corporate, technological culture we sit more at desks and in meetings. What about you? The problem doesn't just plague adults. Too many children no longer play sports and participate in outdoor activities. Instead they get entranced by video games, smartphones, text messages, social networking, online media, TV, and movies. Combined with their favorite fast food, reducing exercise to a flick of the finger on a remote control spells ever-increasing weight gain.

Excessive stress

The excessive stress that most adults and many children labor under also contributes to our expanding waistlines. Stress increases cortisol levels. As a result, many are developing toxic belly fat, thereby increasing their risk for incurring diabetes and other diseases. Long-term stress eventually depletes stress hormones as well as neurotransmitters. This often helps unleash ravenous appetites, plus addictions to sugar and carbohydrates. It's like a nightmarish vortex, each bad habit working to ensnare sufferers in a downward spiral to poor health and disease.

Too much refined sugar and starch

I believe one of the most important reasons for our epidemic of obesity is our high intake of both refined sugars and starches. The standard American diet is full of empty carbohydrates, sugars, fats, excessive proteins, and calories, and it is low in nutrient content. This diet literally causes us to lose nutrients such as chromium, which is crucial in regulating glucose levels in our blood.

The average person consumes 130 pounds of refined sugar per

year.[1] These sugars are sometimes hidden in foods we think are good for us. Take a look at how most of our bread is made. First the outer shell of the grain of wheat is removed. This is the bran or the fiber portion of the grain. The germ of the wheat is then removed; the germ contains the essential fats and vitamin E. These are removed to affect the shelf life of the bread. What is left over is the endosperm, which is the starch of the grain. This is then ground into a very fine powder. The powder of the grain, however, is not white, so it is then bleached with a bleaching agent.

With both the bran and the wheat germ no longer present, and after the bleaching process, very few vitamins remain. Therefore man-made vitamins are then added back, along with sugar, salt, partially hydrogenated fats, and preservatives. White bread is very constipating because it contains no fiber. Also, since it is highly processed when it is consumed, it is rapidly broken down into sugars, and this then causes high amounts of insulin to be secreted, putting a strain on the pancreas and programming our body to store fat.

I believe that increased consumption of white bread, sugar, processed cereals, and pasta is largely responsible for our epidemic of diabetes, high cholesterol, heart disease, and obesity. In centuries past, these refined breads and sugars were given mainly to extremely rich and royal families. This is why many of the wealthy in those days were obese and suffered from diabetes and gout.

A WORD ABOUT WHEAT

The problem with breads, pastas, cereals, and other starches may not be limited to the refining process they undergo. The wheat itself may be the real culprit. Renowned cardiologist William

Davis, MD, believes foods made with or containing wheat are the
number one reason Americans are fat and suffering from diabetes.
Modern wheat strains have been hybridized, crossbred, and
genetically altered by agricultural scientists in order to increase
crop production.[2] As a result, modern strains of wheat have a
higher quantity of genes for gluten proteins that are associated
with celiac disease.[3] Modern wheat also contains a starch called
amylopectin A, which raises blood sugar levels more than virtually
any other carbohydrate.[4]

In addition, wheat is an appetite stimulant, making you want
more and more food.[5] It's also considered addictive. Approximately 30 percent of all people who stop eating wheat products experience withdrawal symptoms such as extreme fatigue,
mental fog, irritability, inability to function at work, and depression.[6] The addictive nature of wheat, coupled with the fact that
it triggers exaggerated blood sugar and insulin responses, sets
your body up to pack on the pounds.

SUGAR AND YOUR BODY

A lot of people think eating fat makes you fat. It's actually the way
your body stores fat that makes you gain weight. Overconsumption
of carbohydrates and sugars stimulates your body's production of
insulin—which is the body's fat storage hormone. Insulin lowers
blood sugar levels when they are too high. However, elevated
insulin levels also cause the body to store fat.

For example, when you eat foods that are high in carbohydrates, such as breads, pasta, potatoes, corn, and rice, the carbohydrate is broken down to glucose, which is absorbed into the
bloodstream. If insulin levels are elevated, the carbohydrate is

more likely to be converted to fat by the liver and then stored away in fat cells.

EASIER ON THAN OFF

If you consume a lot of starch and sugar on a frequent basis, your insulin levels will remain high. If insulin levels remain high, your fat is, figuratively speaking, locked into your fat cells. This makes it very easy to gain weight and extremely difficult to lose weight. Elevated insulin levels usually prevent the body from burning stored body fat for energy. Most obese patients cannot break out of this vicious cycle because they are constantly craving starchy, sugary foods throughout the day, which keeps the insulin levels elevated and prevents the body from burning these stored fats.

> Hear me, O LORD, for Your lovingkindness is good; turn to me according to the multitude of Your tender mercies. And do not hide Your face from Your servant, for I am in trouble; hear me speedily.
> —PSALM 69:16–17

The average person can store about 300–400 grams of carbohydrates in the muscles and about 90 grams in the liver. The stored carbohydrates are actually a stored form of glucose called glycogen. However, once the body storehouses are filled in the liver and muscles, any excess carbohydrates are then usually converted into fat and stored in fatty tissues. When one skips meals or goes over four to five hours without eating, the blood sugar usually decreases, unleashing a ravenous appetite.

Exercise may not help you if you don't eat right. If you eat refined carbohydrates throughout the day, much of the excess carbohydrates will be converted to fat. The high insulin levels also make it more difficult for the body not to release a significant amount of its stored fat. Therefore you can work out for hours at a gym and still not lose fat because you are eating high amounts of carbohydrates and sugar throughout the day. Your body usually will store excess carbohydrates as fat and make it difficult to release any fat that is already stored.

To make matters even worse, when you consume sugar or starches frequently, especially cake, candy, cookies, fruit juices, ice cream, or processed white flour, you may develop low blood sugar within a few hours after eating and unleash a ravenous appetite for more sugar and starch. This raises your blood sugar and your insulin levels, programming you for even more fat storage and preventing you from burning stored fat when you exercise. How frustrating this can be for the uninformed patient. Symptoms of low blood sugar include spaciness, shakiness, irritability, extreme fatigue, headache, sweatiness, racing heart, extreme hunger, or an extreme craving for sweets or starches.

CAUGHT IN A TRAP

This creates a vicious cycle. If you don't eat something sweet or starchy every few hours, you may develop the symptoms of low blood sugar. This is a very important point. You can turn this entire situation around very easily by taking a very simple step: *avoid sugar and refined starches.*

By avoiding sweets, starches, snack foods, junk foods, or high-carbohydrate foods, you can lower your insulin levels and turn off the main trigger that is telling the body to store fat and preventing the body from releasing fat.

When the brain doesn't get enough glucose, you will get cravings. The brain requires a constant supply of glucose. When too much insulin is secreted, such as when you consume a snack that is high in sugar (i.e., a doughnut, a Coke, or cookies), the pancreas then responds by secreting enough insulin to lower the sugar. Often too much insulin is secreted, which lowers the sugar too much, thus causing low blood sugar. Since the brain is not getting the glucose it requires, the low blood sugar creates sugar and carbohydrate cravings, extreme hunger, mood swings, fatigue, and problems concentrating. The brain releases different hormones to increase one's appetite. These signals cause the individual to reach for a sugar or starch "fix" in order to raise the blood sugar the fastest, which will then be able to supply the brain with adequate glucose.

THE POWER OF GLUCAGON

Glucagon is a hormone that works totally opposite than insulin works. Insulin is a fat-storing hormone, whereas glucagon is a fat-releasing hormone. In other words, glucagon will actually enable the body to release stored body fat from the fatty tissues and will permit your muscle tissues to burn your fat as the preferred fuel source instead of blood sugar.

How do you release this powerful substance into your body? It's easy. The release of glucagon is stimulated by eating a correct amount of protein in a meal along with the proper balance of fats and carbohydrates. We will look at this in greater detail later on.

> My flesh and my heart fail; but God is the strength of my heart and my portion forever.
> —PSALM 73:26

When the insulin levels are high in the body, the level of glucagon is low. When glucagon is high, then insulin is low. When you eat a lot of sugar and starch, you raise your insulin levels and lower your glucagon, thus preventing fat from being released to be used as fuel. By simply stabilizing your blood sugar and lowering your insulin levels, you can keep your glucagon levels elevated, which enables your body to burn off the extra fat. Thus you'll begin to realize a more energetic, slimmer you! Eating your protein first helps boost glucagon levels, or you can eat a salad with sliced chicken, turkey, or fish.

SHOULD YOU COUNT CALORIES?

Many people still say, "Why not count calories? A calorie is a calorie." Most people believe that since fat has 9 calories per gram and carbohydrates have only 4 calories per gram, then eating a gram of fat is much more fattening than eating a gram of carbohydrate. But the hormonal effects of fat are not nearly as dramatic as the hormonal effects of carbohydrates and sugars.

Fats will not raise insulin levels, which programs the body to store fat. However, sugars and starches will trigger dramatic releases of insulin, which is the most powerful fat-storing hormone. So don't count calories. Instead, be aware of how your body works. Keep in mind the powerful hormonal effects that sugars and starches have on both insulin, the fat-storing hormone, and on glucagon, the fat-releasing hormone.

The Bible says, "Surely, in vain the net is spread in the sight of any bird" (Prov. 1:17). That means you cannot capture a prey if it understands what's happening. By understanding this powerful truth about how your body actually works, you can avoid the trap of high blood sugar, of high insulin levels, of being overweight or obese, and even of diabetes. Now that you know, the power is in your hands!

GLYCEMIC INDEX 101

The glycemic index was created in the early 1980s to track how quickly insulin levels shot up in individuals after they consumed carbohydrates. While studying individuals with type 2 diabetes, researchers found that certain carbohydrates increased blood sugar levels and insulin levels, while other carbohydrates did not.

They tested hundreds of different foods to determine their glycemic index value. Because their methods and findings have proven so reliable, they are the standard by which we measure the internal processing of foods.

The glycemic index assigns a numeric value to how rapidly the blood sugar rises after consuming a food that contains carbohydrates. Sugars and carbohydrates that are digested rapidly, such as white bread, white rice, and instant potatoes, rapidly increase blood sugar. These are high-glycemic foods and have a glycemic index of 70 or higher. On the other hand, if foods containing carbohydrates are digested slowly and therefore release sugars gradually into the bloodstream, they have a glycemic index value of 55 or lower. These foods include most vegetables and fruits, beans, peas, lentils, sweet potatoes, and the like.

Because these foods cause the blood sugar to rise more slowly, blood sugar levels are stabilized for a longer period of time. Low-glycemic foods also cause satiety hormones to be released in the small intestines, which satisfies you for longer periods of time.

A **BIBLE CURE** Health Fact

Rule of Thumb: The Glycemic Index

Low-glycemic foods: 55 or less

Medium-glycemic foods: 56 to 69

High-glycemic foods: 70 or above

In truth, there is nothing fancy about the glycemic index. One of the most important factors that can determine a food's glycemic index value is to what degree the food has been processed. Generally speaking, the more highly a food is processed, the higher its glycemic index value; the more natural a food, the lower its value.

THE GLYCEMIC LOAD

Almost twenty years after the glycemic index was created, researchers at Harvard University developed a new way of classifying foods that took into account not only the glycemic index value of a food but also the quantity of carbohydrates that particular food contains. This is called the glycemic load (GL). It serves as a guide as to how much of a particular carbohydrate or food we should eat.

For a while nutritionists scratched their heads over patients who wanted to lose weight and were eating low-glycemic foods yet weren't shedding many pounds. Some actually gained weight. Through the GL they discovered that overconsuming many low-glycemic foods can actually lead to weight gain. Not surprisingly, many patients were eating as many low-glycemic foods as they wanted, simply because they had been told that foods with a low value promoted weight loss. They needed to know the whole story, which is how the glycemic load balanced the picture. A food's GL is determined by multiplying the glycemic index value by the quantity of carbohydrates a serving contains (in grams), and then dividing that number by 100. The actual formula looks like this:

- (Glycemic Index Value x Carb Grams per Serving) ÷ 100 = Glycemic Load

To show you how important the GL is, let me offer some examples. Some wheat pastas have a low glycemic index value, which makes many dieters think they're automatically a key to losing weight. However, if a serving size of that wheat pasta is too large, it may sabotage your weight-loss efforts. Despite a low glycemic index value, the pasta's GL is high. Another example is white potatoes, which have a GL double that of yams. On the other end of the scale, watermelon has a high glycemic index value but a very low GL, which makes it OK to eat in a larger quantity.

Don't worry, though. You will not have to calculate the GL for every item you eat. By understanding the GL, you can identify which low-glycemic foods can cause trouble if you eat too much of them. These include low-glycemic breads, low-glycemic rice, sweet potatoes, yams, low-glycemic pasta, low-glycemic cereals, and so forth. As a general rule, any large quantity of a low-glycemic "starchy" food will usually have a high GL.

GLYCEMIC INDEX VALUES OF COMMON FOODS[7]			
Food*	Glycemic Index Value	Food	Glycemic Index Value
Asparagus	15	Broccoli	15
Celery	15	Cucumber	15

GLYCEMIC INDEX VALUES OF COMMON FOODS[7]			
Green beans	15	Low-fat yogurt (artificially sweetened)	15
Peppers (all varieties)	15	Spinach	15
Zucchini	15	Tomatoes	15
Cherries	22	Green peas	22
Black beans	30	Milk (skim)	32
Apples	36	Spaghetti (whole wheat)	37
All-Bran cereal	42	Lentil soup (canned)	44
Orange juice	52	Bananas	53
Potato (sweet)	54	Rice (brown)	55
Popcorn	55	Muesli	56
Whole-wheat bread	69	Watermelon	72
Doughnut	75	Rice cakes	82
Corn flakes	84	Potato (baked)	85
Baguette (French bread)	95	Parsnips	97

* To look up the glycemic index values of other foods not listed above, go to www.thecandodiet.com or http://tinyurl.com/glycemic-index-list.

The amount of fiber in your food, the amount of fat, how much sugar is in the carbohydrates, and proteins all determine the glycemic index score of what you eat.

THREE TYPES OF SUGAR

Three main types of simple sugars (called monosaccharides) make up all carbohydrates. These include:

- Glucose
- Fructose
- Galactose

Glucose is found in breads, cereals, starches, pasta, and grains. Fructose is found in fruits, and galactose is found in dairy products. Plain sugar, or sucrose, is a disaccharide and consists of glucose and fructose joined.

The liver rapidly absorbs these simple sugars. However, only glucose can be released directly back into the bloodstream. Fructose and galactose must first be converted to glucose in the liver to gain entrance into the bloodstream. Thus they are released at a much slower rate. Fructose, found primarily in fruits, has a low glycemic index compared to glucose and galactose.

OTHER GLYCEMIC FOODS

Fiber is a form of carbohydrate that is not absorbed. However, it does slow down the rate of absorption of other carbohydrates. Thus the higher the fiber content of the carbohydrate or starch, the more slowly it will be absorbed and enter the bloodstream. Most fruits are high in fiber and have a low glycemic value. The exceptions are bananas, raisins, dates, and other dried fruits. Almost all vegetables are high in fiber and low-glycemic except for potatoes, carrots, corn, and beets, which have a high glycemic value.

In the next chapter we will discuss in more detail the best foods to eat for overall good health and especially if you want to lose weight. The right carbohydrates balanced with the proper portions of proteins and fats will create a much lower glycemic effect on your body and interrupt the vicious cyle of weight gain.

> I will be glad and rejoice in Your mercy, for You have considered my trouble; You have known my soul in adversities.
>
> —PSALM 31:7

THE WORST KIND OF FAT

You may not like the number on your scale, but that figure does not tell the whole story regarding your overall health. Researchers are finding that one of the greatest indicators of potential health problems is having a high percentage of belly fat. The fat that settles in the belly is different from other types of fat in the body. Fatty tissue or fat storage areas, such as belly fat, are active endocrine organs that produce numerous types of hormones, such as resistin (which increases insulin resistance), leptin (which decreases appetite), and adiponectin (which improves insulin sensitivity and helps to lower blood sugar). The more belly fat cells you have, typically the more estrogen, cortisol, and testosterone your body produces. This is one of the reasons obese men typically develop breasts and obese women often grow hair on their faces. Their fat cells are manufacturing more estrogen and testosterone, respectively.

When your fatty tissues spew out all these hormones—most likely raising your estrogen, testosterone, and cortisol levels—and produce tremendous inflammation in your body, the result is weight gain. Your extra toxic belly fat then sets the stage for type 2 diabetes, heart disease, stroke, cancer, and a host of other diseases. That's because belly fat is like a wildfire. It spreads throughout your body and inflames your cardiovascular system, which eventually causes the production of plaque in your arteries and inflammation in the brain. This can even potentially lead to Alzheimer's disease.

The dangers of this toxic belly fat is one reason this Bible Cure encourages you to set a weight-loss goal based on your waistline rather than your body weight. Typically if your waist measurement increases, your blood sugar will increase; if your waist measurement decreases, your blood sugar will decrease. By reducing your waist measurement, you will probably reverse your risk of many diseases. In fact, lowering waist size ranks higher than weight loss.

Although it is helpful to weigh yourself on a regular basis, I want you to start looking at your waistline as a key indicator of weight management. You should measure your waist around your navel (and love handles, if you have them). Initially your waist measurement goal should be 40 inches or less if you're a man and 35 inches or less if you're a woman. But your ultimate goal should be to have a waist measurement that is half your height or less. For example, a 5-foot-10-inch man is 70 inches tall, so his waist around the belly button and love handles should be 35 inches or less.

OTHER WEIGHT MANAGEMENT MEASURES

While I see waist size as the most important measurement for establishing weight-loss goals, another key measurement is body fat percentage. There are many ways to measure body fat percentage, including a bioimpedance analysis, underwater weighing, and using skinfold calipers. Whatever the method, you need to have your body fat percentage measured the same way each time. Consistency is the key, since the percentage can fluctuate dramatically with inaccurate measurements.

I hold more stock in body fat percentage than I do the body mass index reading. The reason is simple: accuracy. BMI uses only height and weight to judge how overweight or obese a person is. For example, a twenty-three-year-old professional football player and a fifty-six-year-old executive may both be 5 feet 10 inches tall and weigh 220 pounds. This gives both men a BMI of approximately 35, which is considered obese.

In reality, however, the football player can have a 32-inch waist and a remarkable 6 percent body fat; the executive can have a 44-inch waist and 33 percent body fat. That is an astounding 27 percent differential in body fat percentage alone, which the BMI doesn't take into account.

Although many physicians simply use BMI to determine if a person is overweight or obese, I strongly believe more accurate assessments come from using body fat percentage and waist measurements. However, because it is a helpful tool to measure your weight loss goals, I have included the following chart to help you determine your BMI.

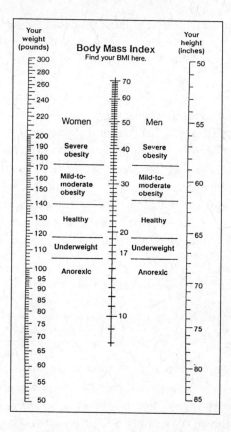

RATING YOUR BODY FAT PERCENTAGE

According to the American Council on Exercise, a body fat percentage greater than 25 percent in men and greater than 33 percent in women is considered obese. A healthy percent body fat in women is 25–31 percent and in men is 18–25 percent.[8]

Initially, obese men should aim for a reading of less than

25 percent, while obese women should shoot for less than 33 percent. Eventually aim for a percent body fat in the healthy range. However, body fat ranks second to your initial focus to reduce your waist measurement.

Many health clubs, nutritionists, and physicians have the equipment to measure your percentage of body fat. Once you have this initial number, monitor it each month.

However, don't get too hung up on body fat or other measurements like your BMI reading. Mainly focus on one thing and one thing only: your waist measurement. You really do not need a scale or any other fancy tools—just a tape measure. By focusing on your waist and achieving your goal measurement, you will eliminate one of the main risk factors for disease.

> His divine power has given to us all things that pertain to life and godliness, through the knowledge of Him who called us by glory and virtue.
> —2 PETER 1:3

If you see yourself in the symptoms I've described in this chapter, don't wait. Make a decision to stop the process of disease in your body right now. God will help you to stay with it if you give Him an opportunity. Why not turn this entire matter over to Him right now? God is at your side to help you. He promises, "I will never leave you nor forsake you" (Heb. 13:5). God is your helper and loves you more than you will ever know. He longs to give you all the strength, power, and hope you need to triumph in your battle. Pray this Bible Cure prayer and keep pressing forward.

A **BIBLE CURE** Prayer for You

*Lord God, You alone are my strength and my source. My
ability to stay committed to weight loss and healthy eating
comes from You. Help me to maintain the willpower I need
to eliminate sugar and empty calories from my diet. Give
me the focus I need to implement all that I am learning.
Almighty God, replace any discouragement with hope and
any doubt with faith. I know that You are with me and
will not leave me. I thank You, Lord, for seeing me through
this battle and giving me victory over obesity. Amen.*

A **BIBLE CURE** *Prescription*

Measure your waistline at your navel; write down the figure: _____

Write down your goal waist measurement: _____

Take a brief self-assessment by answering the following questions.

❑ How many times a day do you eat sugars and carbohydrates?

_____

_____

❑ Describe how you can reduce that frequency.

_____

_____

❑ List the foods high in sugar and starch that you need to eliminate from your diet:

_____

_____

_____

❑ What foods high in protein and fiber can you add to your diet? What high-glycemic foods can you eliminate?

_____

_____

_____

Chapter 2

THE FOUNDATION OF HEALTHY EATING

G OD SKILLFULLY DESIGNED your body as an incredible, living creation that will operate at peak efficiency and health when it is supplied with proper nutrition. In the previous chapter we looked at many of the reasons Americans are obese. Now I want to take a look at the powerful nutritional foundation that will help you to discover a healthier, happier, more attractive you.

CHOOSING THE RIGHT CARBOHYDRATES

Certain carbohydrates are critical for good health. When combined with the correct portions of fats and proteins, good carbs give you energy, calm your mood, keep you full and satisfied by turning off hunger, and assist in weight loss. They also help you to enjoy meals and snacks, enable you to handle stress better, allow you to sleep more soundly, improve your bowel function, and give you an overall feeling of well-being.

However, as with so many things in the land of excess, most Americans have fallen in love with the wrong kind of carbs. They see their waistlines getting wider and wider as a result of eating too much sugar, starch, bread, and pasta, and think the answer is to swear off all carbohydrates. The problem is, high-protein diets are often hard to maintain for long and in some cases they have damaging effects on health. The answer isn't a no-carb diet, but one rich in the right kinds of carbohydrates.

The National Institutes of Health recommends that 45 to 65 percent of daily energy intake for adults come from carbohydrates, with 20 to 35 percent of energy coming from fats, and only 10 to 35 percent from proteins.[1] The American Diabetes Association also recommends 45 to 60 grams of carbohydrates in each meal, preferably from healthy whole grains. I believe this is too many carbohydrates and too much grain. I believe excessive carbohydrates and grains—especially wheat and corn products—are one of the main reasons for our obesity epidemic. I typically recommend about 50 to 55 percent of daily calories come from low-glycemic carbohydrates, 15 to 20 percent from plant and lean animal proteins, and 25 to 30 percent from healthy fats.

Because wheat and corn can trigger exaggerated blood sugar responses, I have my patients give up all wheat and corn products for a season or until they reduce their belly or body fat. Even if breads at the supermarket are called whole-grain breads, they still contain amylopectin A, which usually spikes blood sugar, programming the body for fat storage and weight gain. Therefore if my patients request bread, I recommend that they have small amounts of millet bread in the morning or at lunch. It contains no wheat. However, if weight loss stalls, I have my patients stop eating millet bread. Once a person reaches his goal waist measurement or weight, if he can practice moderation, I have him add back small servings of wheat and corn for breakfast or lunch, but not dinner.

THE TORTOISE AND THE HARE

So how can a person know which are the right carbs to choose? Many people are familiar with the old story about the tortoise and the hare. The hare races ahead but fails to reach the finish line, while the slow but steady tortoise eventually passes him and wins the race. When it comes to how your body processes carbohydrates, the race that takes place within you is reminiscent of this classic fable. I've used these familiar characters to identify two main types of carbohydrates we will talk about in this Bible Cure: low-glycemic "tortoise carbs" and high-glycemic "hare carbs."

> I will love You, O LORD, my strength.
> —PSALM 18:1

Unfortunately most of the carbohydrates overweight and obese people consume are high-glycemic "hare carbs," which cause the blood sugar to rise rapidly. As I have already alluded to, this starts a chain of events that trap people in a fat-storage mode and prevent them from losing weight. The underlying cycle of hare carbs is obvious enough: the faster you absorb the carbs, the higher your insulin level rises, the more weight you gain, and the more diseases you develop. You become literally programmed for weight gain.

When it comes to weight-loss success, "tortoise carbs" are the long-term winners. These are the carbohydrates that slowly raise the blood sugar and enable you to lose weight and prevent or reverse diseases. These low-glycemic tortoise carbs can be broken down into the following groups:

- Vegetables (except potatoes)
- Fruits (except bananas and dried fruits)
- Starches, such as millet bread, brown rice pasta, steel-cut oatmeal, sweet potatoes, new potatoes, brown rice, and wild rice, in small quantities (Minimize these starches; some patients have to eliminate them altogether.)
- Dairy products, such as skim milk; low-fat, low-sugar yogurt; kefir; and low-fat cottage cheese (Minimize dairy products.)
- Legumes, such as beans, peas, lentils, hummus, and peanuts (I recommend 1–4 cups of these starches a day, but start with small servings. You may need Beano, an enzyme that helps you digest beans and minimize gas.)
- Nuts and seeds (raw) (a handful a day)

Even though most of these tortoise carbohydrates are healthy, it's still possible to choose the wrong types of starches and dairy or overeat low-glycemic starches, such as millet bread and brown rice pasta. For this reason, and because there are other ways carbohydrates stall weight-loss efforts, it's important to incorporate the glycemic index and glycemic load principles I discussed in the previous chapter.

> No temptation has overtaken you except such as is common to man; but God is faithful, who will not allow you to be tempted beyond what you are able, but with the temptation will also make the way of escape, that you may be able to bear it.
>
> —1 CORINTHIANS 10:13

IS IT A HARE OR A TORTOISE?

The faster your body digests a carbohydrate, the faster it raises your blood sugar—and the higher the glycemic index value of that carb. This is what makes a carb a hare rather than a tortoise. Yet how exactly can you differentiate between the two? Here are a few traits that will help distinguish between a tortoise and a hare.

Fat content. With the exception of seeds, nuts, and dairy, most tortoise carbohydrates are low in fat. Fats are not an inherent evil, as some diets claim. But consuming highly processed, high-fat carbohydrates will sabotage your weight-loss efforts.

Fiber content. Generally a higher fiber content of a food slows down the absorption of sugar, making the carb a tortoise. Beans, peas, and lentils are high in fiber.

Form of starch. Certain starches, such as potatoes, bread, pasta, and white rice, contain amylopectin, which is a complex carbohydrate that the body rapidly absorbs and that usually raises one's blood sugar. However, beans, peas, legumes, and sweet potatoes contain another complex carb called amylose, which is digested more slowly and raises the blood sugar in a slower fashion. Caution is needed with whole-wheat products, as I have discussed. Almost all corn products are considered hare carbohydrates (with a high glycemic index value). Exceptions are corn on the cob and frozen corn, because they are digested more slowly and gradually raise the blood sugar.

Ripeness. The riper the fruit, the faster it is absorbed. For instance, brown, spotted bananas raise blood sugar much faster than regular yellow bananas since they have a higher sugar content.

Cooking. Most brown rice pasta can be either a tortoise carbohydrate or a hare carbohydrate, depending on how you cook it. If you cook it al dente, still leaving it firm, it is typically a tortoise carbohydrate and has a low glycemic index value. Also, thicker pasta noodles generally have a lower glycemic index value than thinner types of pasta (angel hair, thin spaghetti, etc.). Again, I don't recommend any wheat pasta products, even whole grain, since they have a higher glycemic load than many other carbohydrates.

Milling type. A finely ground grain is a hare carbohydrate and has a higher glycemic index value than coarsely ground grain, which has a higher fiber content and thus is a tortoise.

Protein content. The higher the protein content of a food, the more it helps prevent a rapid rise in blood sugar and makes the food more likely to be lower glycemic. Thus it is a tortoise carbohydrate.

A **BIBLE CURE** Health Tip
PGX Fiber

PGX, short for PolyGlycoPlex, is a unique blend of highly viscous fibers that act synergistically to create a much higher level of viscosity than the individual fibers alone. PGX absorbs hundreds of times its weight in water over one to two hours and expands in the digestive tract, creating a thick gelatinous material. It creates a feeling of fullness, stabilizes blood sugar and insulin levels, and stabilizes appetite hormones.

PGX lowers blood sugar after eating by about 20 percent and lowers insulin secretion by about 40 percent. Researchers have found that higher doses of PGX can decrease appetite significantly. PGX works similar to gastric banding and has fewer gastrointestinal side effects than other viscous dietary fibers. However, start slowly, or you may develop gas.

To aid in weight loss, I recommend starting with two or three capsules of PGX fiber with 16 ounces of water before every meal and gradually increasing the dose if needed. This usually prevents you from overeating and enables you to feel satisfied sooner. (See Appendix B.)

THE POWER OF PROTEIN

Proteins and amino acids are the building blocks for the body. They are used to repair and maintain tissues such as muscles, connective tissue, our skin, our hair, our bone matrix, and even our nails. If you do not have adequate protein, you will not be able to adequately maintain these tissues I just listed, as well as enzymes, hormones, and your immune system. As a result, you will age faster and eventually develop disease.

> Beloved, I pray that you may prosper in all things and be in health, just as your soul prospers.
> —3 JOHN 2

But in the same way too many low-glycemic carbs can sabotage your weight-loss goals, so can too much protein have a negative effect on your well-being. Studies have shown that men with diets high in red meat have an increased risk of prostate cancer, and it is typically a more aggressive form of prostate cancer. However, men who eat fish three times a week have approximately half the risk of developing prostate cancer compared to men who rarely eat fish. Also, frying or grilling meat, chicken, or fish so that it is charred or well done is also associated with an increased risk of cancer.

In 2002 the NIH advised that protein should make up 15 to 35 percent of a person's daily consumption of energy or total calories. I believe that anything more than 35 percent of our daily calories as protein is simply too much. I tell my patients to get approximately 15 to 20 percent of their daily calories from protein, but I recommend only 10 percent or less of our calories should come from animal protein. This usually translates into 3 ounces of animal protein once or twice a day for women and 3 to 6 ounces of animal protein once or twice a day for men. Men should limit red meat to only 12 ounces a week. I also strongly believe in consuming some protein with each meal and snack, but realize that we don't need animal protein with each meal. Beans and a small amount of brown rice (the size of a tennis ball) is a complete protein. This helps to create the correct fuel mixture that keeps your appetite controlled, your energy up, and your blood sugar and insulin levels in check—all while your metabolism continues to burn off those extra pounds.

Free-range or organic lean chicken and turkey; organic or omega-3 eggs; wild-caught, low-mercury fish; and organic low-fat dairy are the best choices of animal proteins. These meats are free of hormones and antibiotics that can be harmful to the body. Also, avoid or limit high-fat junk meats such as hot dogs, bologna, salami, pepperoni, and bacon, which are loaded with salt, nitrates, and nitrites. Nitrates and nitrites are associated with an increased risk of certain cancers.

Organic legumes, whole grains, and nuts are the best plant proteins. Vegetarians are able to combine plant proteins with their regular meals to have a high-quality protein. For example, by combining whole grain rice and beans you can form complete proteins. Soy, however, is an exception and is already considered a complete protein.

The potential problem with combining two starches to make a complete protein is that it is easy to slow down or entirely stop your weight loss if your portions are too big. If you can keep this in mind, however, there is no reason you should not enjoy the added benefits and flavors of these proteins. Black bean soup or lentil soup and a small amount of wild rice is a complete protein and very filling—and yes, you will most likely start losing weight if you regularly consume it.

Plant-based protein powder is also a good way to add protein to your meals and snacks. But you should consume soy products with caution. Many scientists now believe that over-consuming soy may do more harm than good. High consumption of isoflavones, which are the estrogen-like plant chemicals contained in soy, may stimulate the production of breast cancer cells. It may also increase the chances of developing serious reproductive, thyroid, and liver problems.[2]

Besides this, most soy products are processed and have a low biological value compared to other proteins—meaning the body doesn't use them very efficiently. This includes two of the most commonly consumed soy products, soy milk and soy protein. These products can interfere with thyroid function and lower the metabolic rate, making it more difficult to lose weight.

I recommend cutting back on soy products if you desire to lose weight. And let me emphasize this: the final word on soy is not yet in. Even the soy skeptics say the bottom line is to opt for natural forms of soy rather than chemically altered or genetically modified (GM). Because it remains a somewhat controversial protein, my advice is to proceed with caution; do not eat or drink soy products every day, but if you must consume soy, do it only a few times a week.

THE TRUTH ABOUT FAT

Too much of any fat—whether good or bad—will make you fat. But overall, fats are critically important for our health. Among their many roles, their main purpose in the body is to provide fuel for cells. Each of the trillions of cells in your body is surrounded by a fatty cell membrane composed primarily of polyunsaturated and saturated fats. The saturated fats provide a rigid support for the cell membrane. The polyunsaturated fats, meanwhile, add flexibility to the cell membranes and allow the transfer of nutrients inside the cells and waste products to be passed outside the cells. These cell membranes need a proper balance of both saturated and polyunsaturated fats.

Likewise, we need a proper balance of fats in our diet to help with the absorption of fat-soluble vitamins, including vitamins A, D, E, and K. We also need fats to produce hormones that regulate inflammation, blood clotting, and muscle contraction. Approximately 60 percent of your brain is composed of fat. You need cholesterol to make brain cells, and most of your cholesterol comes from saturated fats. Fats make up the coverings that surround and protect nerves. They help to satisfy hunger for extended periods. As you can see, fats are not the villains we have made them out to be.

The majority of Americans consume approximately one-third of their total calories from fats. Even though this is a fairly safe amount of fat, Americans continue to gain weight and suffer from an epidemic of being overweight and obese. For this reason, I recommend approximately 25 to 30 percent of your total calorie intake as fats (making sure to choose *good* fats) in order to lose weight.

Bad fats include trans fats and refined omega-6 fats such as most commercial oils, salad dressings, gravies, sauces, and deep-fried foods. Fats that are good in moderation and fats that are bad in excess include saturated fats and unrefined omega-6 fats such as cold-pressed vegetable oils. Good fats include omega-3 fats such as fish oils, flaxseed, salba seed, hemp and chia seed, and oils made from these seeds; monounsaturated fats such as extra-virgin olive oil, avocados, almonds, and other nuts and seeds; and GLA omega-6 fatty acids such as borage oil, evening primrose oil, and black currant seed oil.

I believe no more than 5 to 10 percent of your fat intake should be saturated fats. I strongly recommend that you avoid all trans fats, deep-fried and pan-fried (not stir-fried) foods, and refined omega-6 fats, such as most regular salad dressings, sauces, and gravies. Consuming modest amounts of omega-3 fats, monounsaturated fats, GLA omega-6 fats, and raw seeds and nuts will help decrease insulin resistance, which in turn enables you to lose weight. Our bodies need the proper balance of good healthy oils for all our cells, tissues, and organs to function properly. Fats are not evil; they're essential.

What you eat makes all the difference in the world for your

overall well-being! Ask God to give you a new way of looking at nutrition. You'll be surprised at the way your thinking about food begins to change.

A **BIBLE CURE** Prayer for You

Lord, I thank You that I am fearfully and wonderfully made. Your Word says we perish for lack of knowledge. Thank You for teaching me about how my body works. Help me to make wise choices so I can lose excess belly fat, be healthy, and function at my best. In Jesus's name, amen.

A **BIBLE CURE** *Prescription*

Take inventory of the foods you typically eat.
• Describe how you will add more good carbohydrates into your diet.

_____

_____

_____

• List the foods that you need to eliminate from your diet:

_____

_____

_____

• Write a prayer asking God to help you choose foods that will allow your body to function at its best and cause you to lose excess fat:

_____

_____

_____

_____

Chapter 3

POWER FOR CHANGE THROUGH DIET AND NUTRITION

W OULD YOU LIKE a supernatural guarantee for success? Here it is: the Bible says to commit your plans to the Lord. "Commit your works to the LORD, and your thoughts will be established" (Prov. 16:3). So I want to encourage you to study this plan and then commit it to the Lord for the strength and willpower to follow through.

God is greater than any bondage you may have. And He promises to help you succeed, not with your own power, but by asking for His. He is so faithful. When you ask Him for help, He promises never to fail you or leave you struggling all alone. For the Word of God says, "For He Himself has said, 'I will never leave you nor forsake you'" (Heb. 13:5). What a powerful promise!

In this chapter we will look at the eating habits that will lead to healthy, consistent weight loss. But first a word of caution. As I have said before, the number on the scale is not the best measure of weight loss. Make sure you keep the right focus. Instead of focusing on how much you weigh, focus on eating right. When you eliminate sugar, sweets, excessive carbohydrates, bad fats, wheat, and corn from your diet, you will most likely begin to lose weight.

This Bible Cure waist-reducing plan is more than a diet. It is a lifestyle that will help you to look and feel your very best. So, let's get started.

THE MEDITERRANEAN DIET

According to a recent study, "People who eat a Mediterranean-style diet rich in fruits, vegetables, whole grains, olive oil, and fish have at least a 25 percent reduced risk of dying from heart disease and cancer."[1] This is because the Mediterranean diet derives roughly 30 to 40 percent of its calories from healthy fats (coming from foods like olive oil, avocados, nuts, and fish) and about 40 to 50 percent from healthy carbohydrates like fruits, vegetables, beans, peas, lentils, and whole grains. Researchers also surmised that it was not any one component of this diet that makes it preventative, but it's the overall combination of foods, as well as avoiding foods that are potentially harmful, such as excessive calories from omega-6 oils, butter, sweets, and meats.

Combined with daily exercise, this is a powerful diet for living a longer and healthier life. Another study estimated that up to 25 percent of the incidence of colorectal cancer, about 15 percent of the incidence of breast cancer, and about 10 percent of the incidence of prostate cancer could be prevented if we shifted from a common Western diet to a traditional Mediterranean one.[2]

I believe the Mediterranean diet should be the foundation of your daily meal-planning, but you will need to make adjustments. Although breads and pastas are staples of the Mediterranean diet, I highly recommend that you avoid wheat and corn products at least until you have reached your desired waist measurement. You will also need to choose foods that do not create an inflammatory response in your body. But before we discuss what foods to avoid, let's first take a look at the primary foods in the Mediterranean diet. (For a more detailed look at the Mediterranean diet, refer to my books *Dr. Colbert's "I Can Do This" Diet*, *Eat This and Live!*, and *What Would Jesus Eat?*)

- *Extra-virgin olive oil*—replaces most fats, oils, butter, and margarine. It is used in salads as well as for cooking. Extra-virgin olive oil strengthens the immune system. I recommend 4 tablespoons a day.

- *Bread*—consumed daily and prepared as whole-grain, dark, chewy, crusty loaves. I recommend waiting until you reach your desired weight or waist size to eat bread. At that point, choose whole- and sprouted-grain breads such as Ezekiel 4:9 bread but avoid white processed bread. (I do not recommend wheat or corn until you have achieved your desired waist measurement.)

- *Thick, whole-grain pasta; brown or wild rice; couscous; bulgur; potatoes*—often served with fresh vegetables and herbs, sautéed in olive oil, and occasionally served with small quantities of lean beef. Again, I recommend avoiding pasta and all wheat products to lose weight. Also, limit the other starches to a tennis-ball serving, but no more than one of these starches a meal.

- *Fruit*—preferably raw, two to three pieces daily, but avoid bananas and dried fruit

- *Nuts*—pecans, almonds, cashews, macadamia nuts, hazelnuts, and walnuts; preferably raw, and one handful a day

- *Beans*—including pintos, great northern, navy, black, red, and kidney beans. Hummus, beans, and lentil soups are very popular (prepared with a small amount of extra-virgin olive oil). I recommend at least 1 to 4 cups of beans, peas, lentils, or hummus a day either as a soup or with the entree. (Beano helps prevent gas.)

- *Vegetables*—all types, including dark green variety, especially in salads, or eaten raw or steamed. Eat a large salad with extra-virgin olive oil and vinegar, and choose romaine, spinach, arugala, etc., but do not choose iceberg lettuce. Iceberg lettuce is very low in fiber and nutritional content. Avoid the croutons.

- *Small amounts of low-fat organic cheese and yogurt*—cheese may be grated on soups or entrees. (The reduced-fat cheeses often taste better than the fat-free varieties. The best yogurt is Greek yogurt, fat free, and organic without added fruit, but not frozen.) Also, try grated feta or goat cheese in place of regular cheese.

In addition to eating the foods listed above, the following foods consumed a few times weekly make a good addition to the Mediterranean diet.

- *Fish.* The healthiest fish are cold-water varieties such as cod, wild salmon, sardines, and tongol tuna. These are high in omega-3 fatty acids. Avoid farm-raised fish and high-mercury fish. (See "Bible Cure Health Fact: Mercury Levels in Fish.")

- *Organic or free-range poultry.* Poultry should be eaten two to three times weekly. Eat white breast meat with the skin removed.

- *Organic or omega-3 eggs.* These should be eaten only in small amounts (two to three per week). I recommend eating only one egg yolk with three egg whites and adding veggies to make an omelet once or twice a week and cooked in extra-virgin olive oil.

- *Organic or free-range lean red meat.* Red meat should be eaten only rarely, on an average of once or twice a week. (I suggest consuming less than 12 ounces of red meat a week.) Use only lean cuts with the fat trimmed. Use in small amounts as an additive to spice up soup or pasta. (Note: the severe restriction of red meat in the Mediterranean diet is a radical departure from the American diet, but it is a major contributor to the low rates of cancer, heart disease, and stroke found in these countries.)

A **BIBLE CURE** Health Fact
Dueling Diets

A study published by the *New England Journal of Medicine* found that following a Mediterranean-style diet helped participants reduce their risk of heart attack, stroke, and death from heart disease by 30 percent. In fact, the benefits of the Mediterranean diet on heart health were so clear, the study was stopped early. Conducted in Spain, the study randomly assigned more than 7,000 people who had various risk factors for heart disease including obesity and diabetes to one of three groups. One group followed a low-fat diet, and two groups were put on a Mediterranean diet, eating fish, grains, fruits, and vegetables while avoiding red meats and processed foods. One of the groups assigned to the Mediterranean diet was instructed to eat at least 4 tablespoons of extra-virgin olive oil a day and the other an ounce—or roughly a quarter cup—of walnuts, hazelnuts, and almonds each day. Not only did those on the Mediterranean diet lower their heart disease risk, but they were also able to stay with the diet. The low-fat dieters were not able to stick with the plan and ended up eating a typical modern diet.[3]

A DEADLY BY-PRODUCT OF THE WESTERN DIET: INFLAMMATION

One of the biggest problems with our modern, high-fat, highly processed, high-sugar, high-grain (such as wheat and corn), high-sodium diets is that it has thrown off the balance in our bodies between inflammatory and anti-inflammatory chemicals called *prostaglandins*. Normally inflammation is a good thing that works to repair an injury or fight off infection in the body. It puts the immune system on high alert to attack invading bacteria or viruses to rid our body of these intruders, or in the case of an injury, it rushes white blood cells to the cut, scrape, sprain, or broken bone to remove the damaged cells, splint the injury, or attack infections to facilitate healing.

> Who gives food to all flesh, for His mercy endures forever. Oh, give thanks to the God of heaven! For His mercy endures forever.
>
> —PSALM 136:25–26

This is the good side of inflammation and an extremely important function of the immune system's small agents. When our bodies are in such an emergency, there is a complicated process through which more pro-inflammatory prostaglandins are created than anti-inflammatory ones, and the immune system responds to the sounding of this alarm. When the crisis is over, the balance swings in the anti-inflammatory direction and eventually balances out again.

If you look at this process in a grossly simplified sense, you will see that prostaglandins are produced from the foods we eat in an ongoing cycle, and each of the foods we eat has either a pro-inflammatory tendency or an anti-inflammatory one. Fatty acids are at the center of this. Omega-6 fatty acids are "friendly" to the creation of pro-inflammatory prostaglandins, and omega-3 fatty acids are "friendly" to the creation of anti-inflammatory prostaglandins. A more natural, Mediterranean-type diet will have a balance of pro- and anti-inflammatory-friendly foods; however, our modern high-fat, high-sodium, high-sugar, highly processed

Western diet throws that balance off in favor of the production of pro-inflammatory prostaglandins.

Experts tell us that our typical US diet has doubled the amount of omega-6 fatty acids we consume since 1940 as we have shifted more and more away from fruits and vegetables to grain-based foods and the oils produced from them. In fact, we eat about twenty times more omega-6s than we do the anti-inflammatory omega-3s. Most of the animals we obtain food from today are also grain fed, so most of our meats, eggs, and dairy products are higher in omega-6s than they were a century ago. Also, as most of the fish in our stores are now farm raised, they are fed a diet of cereal grains instead of the algae and smaller fish they would live on in the wild, so even our fish are more sources of omega-6s than they used to be. Noting all of this, it is not hard to see why diseases caused by chronic systematic inflammation have grown to be such a problem in the Western world today.

Furthermore, essential fatty acids (EFAs) such as omega-3 and omega-6 cannot be manufactured in the body and must be consumed either through diet or supplements. EFAs help the body repair and create new cells. In addition to reducing inflammation, omega-3 fatty acids can actually create special roadblocks in the body, making it harder for cancer cells to migrate from a primary tumor to start new colonies. Cancers that remain localized in one place are much easier to treat than those that metastasize (spread throughout the body).[4]

Because of the high omega-6 content of our diets, our bodies find more material for pro- than anti-inflammatory prostaglandins. Over time the natural, ongoing creation of prostaglandins will tip the balance toward systematic inflammation as more pro-inflammatory prostaglandins are produced than anti-inflammatory ones. Despite the absence of an actual emergency, this imbalance still sets off alarms calling for chronic or long-term inflammation, and the immune system will respond accordingly. However, with no actual threat present, the immune system will start attacking things it normally wouldn't. This immune hypersensitivity can lead to a glut of problems ranging from simple allergies and weight gain to cancer, Alzheimer's disease, cardiovascular disease, diabetes, arthritis, asthma, prostate problems, and autoimmune diseases.

Many of these happen because as the immune system stays on high alert longer than it should, its agents begin to fatigue and make bad decisions, possibly leading to autoimmune disease or not destroying mutated cells, leading to cancer formation with more frequency. This can easily give way to cancer getting a foothold it won't easily relinquish.

> And my God shall supply all your need according to His riches in glory by Christ Jesus.
> —PHILIPPIANS 4:19

Omega-3 fatty acids are clearly incredibly beneficial. Here are some omega-3 foods to include in your diet: flaxseeds and flaxseed oil, chia seeds, salba seeds, hemp seeds, fish (wild salmon, sardines, tongol tuna, herring, and cod), and fish oil. (See Bible Cure Health Fact: Mercury Levels in Fish.) Obviously, it's important to know which fats to eat and which ones to avoid when it comes to preventing those harmful prostaglandins I mentioned above.

So, while using an understanding of the Mediterranean diet as a foundation, within that framework you should also look at how pro-inflammatory or anti-inflammatory the foods you eat are as well. If you are having problems with allergies, joint pains, muscle aches, or the like, by eating more anti-inflammatory foods than pro-inflammatory ones, you can tip your balance back in the right direction.

One way to check your degree of inflammation is to have a C-reactive protein blood test. C-reactive protein is a promoter of inflammation and also a blood marker of systemic inflammation. Once you reach forty years of age, annual CRP testing is a great idea for checking the anti-inflammatory effectiveness of your diet. Men should aim for a CRP less than 1.0, while women should aim for a CRP less than 1.5.

A BIBLE CURE *Health Fact*
Mercury Levels in Fish

Although fish is generally a good protein choice, some fish contain high levels of mercury. The following list will help you determine which fish to eat more liberally and which to avoid.[5]

Fish with least amounts of mercury (enjoy these fish)

- Anchovies
- Catfish
- Crab
- Flounder
- Haddock (Atlantic)
- Herring
- Salmon (fresh or canned)
- Sardines
- Shrimp
- Sole
- Tilapia
- Trout (freshwater)
- Whitefish

Fish with moderate amounts of mercury (eat six servings or less per month)

- Bass (striped or black)
- Halibut (Atlantic or Pacific)
- Lobster
- Mahi-Mahi
- Monkfish
- Snapper
- Tuna (canned, chunk light)

Fish high in mercury (eat three servings or less per month)

- Bluefish
- Grouper
- Mackerel (Spanish and Gulf)
- Sea bass (Chilean)
- Tuna (canned albacore)
- Tuna (yellowfin)

Fish highest in mercury (avoid)

- Mackerel (king)
- Marlin
- Orange roughy
- Shark
- Swordfish
- Tilefish
- Tuna (bigeye and ahi)

THE ANTI-INFLAMMATORY DIET: TAKING THE MEDITERRANEAN DIET TO THE NEXT LEVEL

Using the Mediterranean diet as the foundation for your day-in, day-out meal planning, you can then balance your pro-inflammatory and anti-inflammatory foods as your body (and CRP tests if you have taken them) indicates that you should. This will, of course, initially probably mean adding more anti-inflammatory foods and avoiding the pro-inflammatory ones for a time.

I have organized the following two lists of foods for you to consider adding or subtracting from your diet as your level of systematic inflammation demands.

TOP ANTI-INFLAMMATORY FOODS (ALWAYS CHOOSE ORGANIC WHEN POSSIBLE)	
Fruit	Raspberries, acerola (West Indian) cherries, guava, strawberries, cantaloupe, lemons/limes, rhubarb, kumquat, pink grapefruit, mulberries, blueberries, blackberries
Vegetables	Chili peppers, onions (including scallions and leeks), spinach, greens (including kale, collards, and turnip and mustard greens), sweet potatoes, carrots, garlic
Legumes	Lentils, green beans, peas
Egg products	Liquid eggs, egg whites (may use one organic or free-range egg yolk with three egg whites)
Dairy (use with caution)	Cottage cheese (low fat and nonfat), nonfat cream cheese, plain low-fat Greek yogurt or vanilla Greek yogurt (add fresh fruit if desired) (Limit dairy to 4–6 oz. every three to four days)
Fish	Herring, haddock, wild salmon (not farmed; Alaskan preferred), rainbow trout, sardines, anchovies (See Bible Cure Health Fact: Mercury Levels in Fish.)
Poultry	Goose, duck, free-range organic chicken and turkey (white meat preferred, skins removed) (3–6 oz. once or twice a day)
Meat	Eye of round (beef), flank steak, sirloin tip, skirt steak, pork tenderloin (free range preferred, extra lean or lean) (Limit to 3–6 oz. two times a week, 12 oz. max.)
Cereal	Steel-cut oatmeal, oat bran

Fats/oils	Safflower oil (high oleic), hazelnut oil, extra-virgin olive oil, avocado oil, almond oil, apricot kernel oil
Nuts/seeds	Brazil nuts, macadamia nuts, hazelnuts, pecans, almonds, hickory nuts, cashews (best raw)
Herbs/spices	Garlic, onion, cayenne, ginger, turmeric, chili peppers, chili powder, curry powder, rosemary, boswellia
Sweeteners	Stevia, tagatose, coconut palm sugar
Beverages	Black, white, or green tea, club soda/seltzer, herbal tea, spring water
Starches	Sweet potatoes, new potatoes, millet bread, brown and wild rice, brown rice pasta, and legumes (see above for approved legumes)

INFLAMMATORY FOODS TO LIMIT OR AVOID	
Fruit	Mango, banana, dried apricots, dried apples, dried dates, canned fruits, raisins
Vegetables	White potatoes, french fries, potato chips
Legumes	Baked beans, fava beans (boiled), canned beans
Egg products	Duck eggs, goose eggs, hard-boiled eggs, egg yolks
Cheeses	Brick cheese, cheddar cheese, Colby cheese, cream cheese (normal and reduced fat)
Dairy	Fruited yogurt, ice cream, butter
Fish	Farm-raised fish and fish high in mercury (See Bible Cure Health Fact: Mercury Levels in Fish.)
Poultry	Turkey (dark meat), Cornish game hen, chicken giblets, chicken liver
Meat	Bacon, veal loin, veal kidney, beef lung, beef kidney, beef heart, beef brain, pork chitterlings, lamb rib chops, dark turkey meat with skin, turkey wing with skin, all processed meats

Breads	Hot dog/hamburger buns, English muffins, Kaiser rolls, bagels, french bread, Vienna bread, blueberry muffins, oat bran muffins
Cereal	Grape-Nuts, Crispix, Corn Chex, Just Right, Rice Chex, corn flakes, Rise Krispies, Raisin Bran, shredded wheat
Pasta/grain	White rice, lasagna noodles, macaroni elbows, regular pasta, all corn products except corn on the cob or frozen corn (non-GMO)
Fats/oils	Margarine, wheat germ oil, sunflower oil, poppy seed oil, grape seed oil, safflower oil, cottonseed oil, palm kernel oil, corn oil
Sweeteners	Honey, brown sugar, white sugar, corn syrup, powdered sugar
Crackers/chips/cookies	Corn chips, pretzels, graham crackers, saltines, vanilla wafers
Desserts	Sweetened condensed milk, angel food cake, chocolate and vanilla cake with frosting, chocolate chips, heavy whipping cream, ice cream, fruit leather snacks (Most all desserts are made with sugar.)
Candy	Hershey Kisses, jelly beans, Twix, Almond Joy, milk chocolate bars, Snickers
Beverages	Milk, Gatorade, pineapple juice, orange juice, cranberry juice, lemonade, sodas, sugar-laden soft drinks

These are not complete lists by any means—just some of the more likely "suspects" to watch out for and some of the more helpful helpers to work into your diet. As you read these now, some of them will jump out at you as things you like and need, but you don't have as much of them in your diet as you probably should. Others are the foods that it is time to change your habits about and say good-bye to. The thing to remember is that you have a choice about what you put in your mouth, and now that you have a little more knowledge about these foods, you can begin making healthier diet choices concerning them.

If you have no health problems or obesity, avoiding the inflammatory foods on the previous pages is a good general guideline, and simply follow the Mediterranean diet I outlined earlier. Because your health is good, you have a little more freedom than someone who is struggling with his or her health or weight. You may eat some of the inflammatory foods listed, but I highly recommend you use moderation when consuming them.

> I will instruct you and teach you in the way you should go; I will guide you with My eye.
>
> —PSALM 32:8

If you have health problems or obesity, then in addition to understanding the anti-inflammatory and inflammatory food lists on the previous pages, I advise you to adhere to the following anti-inflammatory diet exactly as directed below and avoid all inflammatory foods. Once your health conditions clear up or you are able to maintain a healthy weight, you can ease up on the following guidelines. If you reintroduce wheat into your diet, choose whole-grain breads and sprouted breads such as Ezekiel 4:9 bread, and avoid white processed bread. But again use moderation whenever eating inflammatory foods.

DR. COLBERT'S ANTI-INFLAMMATORY DIET (ALWAYS CHOOSE ORGANIC WHEN POSSIBLE)	
Vegetables	• Steam, stir fry, or cook under low heat. • Best cooked with extra-virgin olive oil, macadamia nut oil, or coconut oil • Vegetable soups should be non-cream-based, low sodium (homemade is best); you may add some organic meat. • Juice your own vegetable juice; avoid store-bought juices, which are usually high in sodium.
Animal proteins (meat)	• 3 oz. once or twice a day for women; 3 to 6 oz. once or twice a day for men • Wild salmon, sardines, anchovies, tongol tuna, turkey (skin removed), free-range chicken (skin removed), eggs (omega-3 eggs as well) • When grilling, slice meat into thin slices; marinate in red wine, pomegranate juice, cherry juice, or curry sauce. Remove all char from meat. • Be cautious with egg yolks, keeping to a maximum of once or twice a week. You can combine one yolk with two to three egg whites. • Limit consumption of lean beef and red meat to one to two 3 to 6 oz. servings a week.
Fruits	• Berries, Granny Smith apples, lemon, or lime. If diabetic, choose only berries.
Nuts and seeds	• All raw nuts and seeds are acceptable, but just a handful once or twice a day.

Salads	• Use 1-calorie-per-spray salad spritzers; or create your own vinaigrette spritzer using a one to two ratio of extra-virgin olive oil to balsamic, apple cider, or red wine vinegar. So you would mix 1 to 2 Tbsp. extra-virgin olive oil with 2 to 4 Tbsp. vinegar. Once you attain a healthy weight and waistline, increase your olive oil to 4 Tbsp. a day in your salad dressing.
Dairy	• Low-fat dairy without sugar such as Greek yogurt and low-fat cottage cheese
Starches	• Sweet potatoes, new potatoes, brown/wild rice, millet bread, brown rice pasta • Two to four cups daily of beans, peas, legumes, lentils, or hummus • Use moderation when choosing starches, at most only one serving per meal, and make them the size of a tennis ball, not a basketball. • If diabetic, I recommend that you avoid starches.
Beverages	• Alkaline water or sparkling water; may add lemon or lime • Green, black, or white tea; may add lemon or lime • Coffee • Low-fat coconut milk or almond milk in place of cow's milk • No sugar; use stevia or other sugar substitutes such as Just Like Sugar, Sweet Balance, xylitol, chicory, or tagatose or coconut palm sugar in moderation. • No cream; use low-fat coconut milk.

Avoid	• Avoid all gluten (wheat, barley, rye, spelt); this includes all products made with these grains, including bread, pasta, crackers, bagels, pretzels, most cereals, etc. Go to www.celiacsociety.com for gluten-free foods. Also avoid corn products except for corn on the cob. Choose non-GMO.
Avoid	• Inflammatory animal proteins such as shellfish, pork, lamb, veal, and organ meats • Sugar • Fried foods • Processed foods • High-glycemic foods such as white rice, instant potatoes, etc.

Be sure to rotate your vegetables and meats every four days if you have food sensitivities. Do not eat the same food every day.

A BIBLE CURE *Health Fact*

Choose Olive Oil Wisely

Do not buy extra-virgin olive oil packaged in a large plastic bottle. Olive oil is perishable, or it turns rancid. You should buy small amounts, packaged in dark glass bottles, and store it in a dark pantry at a cool temperature. Check expiration dates, and throw it away if it smells or tastes rancid.

A WORD ABOUT PORTION SIZES

Any plan to lose weight will require you to limit your portions, but that doesn't mean you have to feel deprived. Barbara Rolls, PhD, introduced the concept of "volumetrics" as an answer to dieters who were sick of always feeling hunger. Her premise is simple: rather than eating tiny amounts of calorie-dense foods, eat lots of low-calorie foods that are naturally rich in water and fiber. Instead of bothering with counting calories or grams of fat, protein, or carbs, Rolls argues that dieters can eat more than they normally do and still lose weight—as long as they eat the right type of foods (ones that aren't calorie-dense).

Though I differ on many of her points, I believe Rolls is onto something by understanding that you can eat large portions of foods with little to no calories. Vegetables are a perfect example of this, which is why in this Bible Cure program you are essentially able to eat as many vegetables as you want with meals (minus the butter, of course). In fact, there are a few simple volumetric tips you can use at every meal.

- Before every meal drink a tall glass of water with two or three capsules of PGX fiber. This usually prevents you from overeating.

- Enjoy a bowl of vegetable soup, minestrone soup, black bean soup, lentil soup, or any other broth-based, low-sodium, non-cream-based vegetable soup. A study done at Penn State concluded that eating a bowl of soup with an entree actually reduced the total consumed calories by 20 percent.[6] A cup of bean, pea, or lentil soup before your meal is very filling and will help you lose weight, but eat no more than four cups of beans, peas, and lentils per day.

- Precede your entree with a salad (any size). Make sure you use a salad spritzer with 1 calorie per spray. If you decide to eat your salad with extra-virgin olive oil and vinegar, be sure to limit your olive oil to 1 to 2 tablespoons and two or three times as much vinegar. You will use less if you use a salad spritzer. Avoid the croutons.

• Whether eating a salad or your entree, always remember to chew every bite twenty to thirty times; this not only helps your body digest and absorb the food's nutrients, but it also causes you to eat slower and fill up faster.

By prefilling your stomach with low-calorie foods, you are less likely to eat excess amounts of starches, meats, fats, and desserts.

SNACKING RIGHT

Ideally, you should eat every three to three and a half hours to avoid hunger. Many people do not understand that a good snack can turn off your appetite and can stop the triggers from setting it off in the first place. And though it seems counter-intuitive to some, snacking can help you burn more calories in the process. Researchers have determined that snacking on the right amount of healthy foods, in addition to eating three meals a day, boosts the metabolic rate more than if you only eat three meals each day.[7]

The best type of snack food is a mini-meal consisting of healthy protein; a high-fiber, low-glycemic carbohydrate or starch; and some good fat. When mixed together, this food fuel or fuel mixture is digested slowly, causing glucose to trickle into your bloodstream, which controls your hunger for hours. Portion control is a key to wise snacking. Select half a serving of either a low-glycemic starch or one serving size of fruit. Then add 1 to 2 ounces of a protein and a third of a serving size of healthy fat. Typically this mini-meal should amount to just 100 to 150 calories for women and 150 to 250 calories for men. Here are a few examples of well-rounded snacks.

Morning or afternoon snack

- 2 tablespoons of guacamole or avocado with raw carrots or celery
- 2 tablespoons of hummus with raw carrots or celery (4 inches in length)
- 10–15 baked lentil chips and 2 tablespoons of hummus, guacamole, or avocado (You can purchase the baked lentil chips at www .mediterraneansnackfoods.com.)
- 1 to 2 wedges of Laughing Cow Light cheese, 1 ounce of smoked salmon or tongol tuna (meat optional)
- Half a cup of nonfat cottage cheese, a piece of low-glycemic fruit (berries or Granny Smith apple), and 5 to 10 nuts
- A small salad with 1 to 2 ounces of sliced turkey and 2 tablespoons of avocado; use a salad spritzer or 1 tablespoons extra-virgin olive oil mixed with 2 to 3 tablespoons vinegar in a salad spritzer (meat optional)
- A bowl of broth-based vegetable, lentil, or bean soup with 1 to 2 ounces of boiled chicken

- A protein smoothie made from plant protein powder (1–2 scoops) mixed with 2 to 4 ounces of frozen berries and 8 ounces of low-fat coconut or almond milk, or coconut kefir (option: dilute the coconut milk, almond milk, or kefir by reducing it to 4 ounces and combining with 4 ounces of filtered water or spring water)

Evening snacks

- Protein drink
- Lettuce wraps
- Salad with or without lean meat (may use a salad spritzer or one part extra-virgin olive oil mixed with two to three parts vinegar)
- Vegetable or bean or lentil soup with or without lean meat

Be sure to take two or three PGX fiber capsules with a 16-ounce glass of water with your snack. And remember you can add as many non-starchy vegetables as you want. To top it off, I recommend a cup of green or black tea, using natural stevia as a sweetener.

> "Not by might nor by power, but by My Spirit," says the LORD of hosts.
>
> —ZECHARIAH 4:6

Keep plenty of healthy snack items at home, at work, and on the road. Always be prepared. And don't forget: it is important to get snacks that you truly enjoy. Otherwise you won't bother.

A BIBLE CURE *Health Fact*
Timely Eating

Research has shown that people who successfully lose weight and keep it off eat breakfast every day. Other studies have gone a step further, proving that people who skip breakfast are prone to eating more food and snacks during the day.[8]

Unfortunately, most Americans have their meals backward. We skimp on breakfast, eat a medium-size lunch, and then pig out come dinnertime. We should actually be doing the opposite. We should eat breakfast like a king (within thirty minutes of waking up), lunch like a prince, and dinner like a pauper.

Eat every three to three and a half hours to avoid hunger. Eating at the right times will leave you energized, mentally sharper, and more emotionally stable. Even your job performance will go up as a result.

ACCELERATING YOUR WEIGHT LOSS

For those who need to quickly lose weight to ward off or reverse obesity-related illness such as diabetes, I developed the Rapid Waist Reduction Diet. This plan is based on protocol Dr. A. T. W. Simeons developed more than sixty years ago. He found that when his 500-calorie-a-day, very low-fat and very low-carbohydrate diet was combined with small daily doses of the pregnancy hormone hCG (human chorionic gonadotropin), it caused the body to release abnormal collections of fat in the problem areas of the hips, thighs, buttocks, waist, and belly.

In Dr. Simeons's day patients were hospitalized for in-patient treatment for the entire six-week duration of the program. According to Dr. Simeons, 60 to 70 percent of the patients kept the weight off long-term.

Many consider Dr. Simeons's protocol the best-kept medical secret as well as the most effective weight-loss program of all time. In 2007 consumer advocate Kevin Trudeau made Dr. Simeons's protocol known to the world in his book *The Weight Loss Cure "They" Don't Want You to Know About*. I started recommending the Simeons Protocol and monitoring patients back in 2008. At that time I used hCG injections. However, now I recommend either the sublingual hCG tab that is compounded by a compounding pharmacy or homeopathic hCG drops.*

The Food and Drug Administration (FDA) requires us to inform patients of the following statement: "hCG has not been demonstrated to be an effective adjunctive therapy in the treatment of obesity. There is no substantial evidence that it increases weight loss beyond that resulting from calorie restriction, that it causes a more attractive or 'normal' distribution of fat or that it decreases the hunger and discomfort associated with calorie restricted diets."

---

* As of the printing of this book, the FDA does not allow over-the-counter (OTC) hCG drops to be labeled as homeopathic and make claims about weight loss. It is extremely difficult to get homeopathic hCG drops due to the new FDA regulations The drops I recommend have been modified to comply with the FDA. The prescription sublingual hCG tabs I recommend also comply with the FDA restrictions as they are prescribed and not OTC and this new regulation does not pertain to the prescription sublingual hCG drops.

I have modified the 500 calories in the Simeons Protocol to approximately 1,000 calories in my Rapid Waist Reduction Diet, but I've kept Simeons's ratio of proteins, fats, and carbohydrates the same. I also added more soluble fiber and supplements to boost serotonin levels and help with satiety, blood sugar control, and improved bowel movements. Results vary from person to person, but a number of my patients have been able to come off all their medications after following the Rapid Waist Reduction Diet and losing belly fat.

This program is not for everyone. Women who are breastfeeding, pregnant, or planning to become pregnant; those who recently had surgery or cancer; and individuals who have been diagnosed with heart failure, type 1 diabetes, chronic renal failure, severe anemia, mental illness, or any seizure disorders should not participate in this diet plan. Those taking diuretics, anti-inflammatory medications, Coumadin, insulin, or birth control may also be unable to participate.

I believe that anyone should talk with their health care provider before beginning a strict diet or exercise program, but those who are prediabetic or diabetic *must* involve their physicians to ensure the steps they take to incorporate the principles in the Rapid Waist Reduction Diet will work with their particular health needs. If you think this diet is right for you, I encourage you to get my book *The Rapid Waist Reduction Diet,* in which I outline this plan in its entirety.

DON'T GIVE UP

You may think it's impossible for you to lose weight, but with God's help you will get to your goal weight and stay there. Instead of focusing on your weight, focus on the lifestyle and dietary changes you need to make. And don't allow yourself to get stuck thinking you will never succeed at weight loss. Start every day with prayer to God for success. Speak aloud the Bible verses that are scattered throughout this book. In addition, plan your menu each day. With a little patience, you'll be well on your way to becoming the slimmer, healthy person God intended you to be!

A **BIBLE CURE** Prayer for You

Lord, give me the will and determination to eat right and lose weight. Break the bondage of obesity in my life that keeps me from enjoying an abundant life in Christ. Let me be filled with Your strength and power to follow a healthy lifestyle and eat the right foods so that I may serve and love You with my whole heart. Amen.

A **BIBLE CURE** *Prescription*
Keep a Daily Food Diary

Researchers say that self-monitoring devices, such as a pedometer, heart rate monitor, or even a simple exercise journal, can account for a 25 percent increase in successfully controlling your weight.[9] I encourage you to keep a food journal to monitor your waist measurement, your body fat percentage, what you eat, and to log how often you exercise. I have included a sample food diary. Make copies as needed.

To boost your efforts, find a photograph of yourself at or near a healthy or desired weight and put it in your food journal. As you carry your food journal (see below for a sample) with you throughout the day and look at the picture, visualize yourself becoming that ideal weight again. Confession helps too; each day confess that, by faith, you weigh your desired weight.

Date/Weight and Waist Size	Breakfast	Lunch	Dinner

Chapter 4

TIPS FOR EATING OUT

THE NATIONAL RESTAURANT Association estimates Americans spend 49 percent of their food budget at restaurants.[1] With America's fast-paced lifestyle, many parents feel they do not have time to prepare family meals, leading to an unhealthy reliance on fast-food restaurants. Meanwhile singles or couples without children at home have discovered that eating out regularly is easier and may be more economical. I don't recommend that you eat out all the time, but all of us will eat out from time to time—it is part of modern life.

The good news is that you can eat out and still enjoy a balanced, healthy meal. Most restaurants serve unhealthy food, so you can't eat just anything. In addition, portion sizes are often distorted. If you hope to control your weight, there are basic principles you must understand when deciding what dishes to order at restaurants.

- Choose sparkling water or unsweetened tea with a wedge of lemon or lime.
- Take two to four PGX fiber capsules with 16 ounces of unsweetened tea or water to help prevent overeating.
- Avoid the bread. If possible, ask that it not even be placed on the table.

- Choose an appetizer with vegetables and meats such as a shrimp cocktail. Avoid any that are deep-fried, high in starch and fats (i.e., quesadillas or corn bread), or bread based.

- Order your salad with the dressing on the side and with no croutons, cheese, or fattening side items. It's best to bring your own salad dressing spritzer or use olive oil and vinegar.

- Add a bowl of broth-based vegetable or bean or lentil soup to fill yourself up before the entrée.

- Choose entrées with meat, fish, or poultry that is baked, broiled, grilled, or stir-fried in a minimum amount of oil. Avoid anything deep fried or pan-fried. Meat portion sizes should be 3 ounces for women and 3 to 6 ounces for men. If the portion is larger, ask the server to put half in a to-go box.

- Limit sauces and gravies. If you must have them, ask that they be put on the side.

- Ask that vegetables be steamed without butter or oils (unless you prefer them raw).

- Choose sweet potato over white potato when possible. Because these are high-glycemic foods, keep portion to the size of a tennis ball.

- If you choose a dessert, share it and only take a few bites. Savor those bites.

One of the easiest ways to avoid sabotaging your weight-loss goals is planning. This will help you avoid unhealthy foods and overeating. Never go out to eat when you feel ravenous. I guarantee that you will eat too much of the wrong foods. Have a healthy snack such as a large Granny Smith apple or a pear before leaving the house. This will pre-fill your stomach and help prevent overeating.

In addition, plan what and where you will eat before leaving home. I also suggest patients plan an early dinner, usually between five and six o'clock, so they will finish early enough to burn off some calories before going to bed. You may also want to consider sharing an entrée with your spouse. Also, be sure to slow down while eating, and chew every bite thoroughly, putting your fork down between bites. All these "little" things go a long way in controlling hunger and weight.

SPECIALITY RESTAURANTS

Here are some additional tips to help you make wise choices when eating out at specialty food restaurants.

> But the fruit of the Spirit is love, joy, peace, longsuffering, kindness, goodness, faithfulness, gentleness, self-control.
>
> —GALATIANS 5:22–23

Fast-food restaurants

Choose a grilled chicken sandwich or a small hamburger. Throw away the top and bottom bun, and squeeze your burger between two napkins to remove excess grease. Cut the hamburger in half and then place both halves of the meat between two lettuce leafs. Avoid mayonnaise and ketchup; choose mustard, tomato, onions, and pickle. You can also order a small salad and ask for fat-free dressing (or use just a small portion of a regular packet). For a drink, order unsweetened iced tea or a bottle of water. Instead of french fries, order a baked potato when available, using only one pat of butter or 2 teaspoons of sour cream.

If you eat at a sub shop, choose turkey, lean roast beef, and chicken instead of bologna, pastrami, salami, corned beef, or other fatty selections. Choose a 6-inch sub, eating it with the smaller bottom of the bun and not the top portion. Use plenty of vegetables, and top with vinegar; avoid or go easy on the oil. It's best to further cut calories by ordering it in a lettuce or pita wrap.

At fast-food chicken restaurants, choose rotisserie or baked chicken instead of fried. Peel off the skin and pat the chicken dry with a napkin. Drain the liquid from the coleslaw, and do not eat the biscuit or potatoes.

Before diving into a slice of pizza, eat a large salad. Then have only one slice of pizza, sticking to thin or flatbread crust. Choose chunky tomatoes and other veggies as toppings. Avoid pepperoni and other highly processed meat toppings, and ask for half the cheese (the same way many ask for double cheese). Finally, use a napkin to remove excess oils from the cheese.

Italian restaurants

Start with a soup—minestrone, pasta fagioli, or broth-based tomato—and a large salad. Limit bread and olive oil, which has 120 calories per tablespoon. Good entrée options include grilled chicken, fish, shellfish, veal, and steak. Avoid fried or Parmesan dishes, such as chicken or veal Parmesan. Ask for your vegetables to be steamed, and avoid the pasta or have it cooked al dente, which causes it to have a lower glycemic index value. Don't overdo it on the pasta; the amount should be about the size of a tennis ball. Avoid fat-filled creamy sauces, cheese, and pesto sauce.

Mexican restaurants

Avoid the deep-fried tortilla chips, and choose tortilla soup without the chips or black bean soup as appetizers. Be wary of entrées smothered in melted cheese, which automatically increases the fat count. Choose fajitas with chicken, beef, or shrimp. Avoid the tortilla, and make your fajita with lettuce wraps. Add such ingredients as salsa, onions, lettuce, beans, and guacamole. Avoid cheese and sour cream if possible, since restaurants rarely serve nonfat varieties. As for beans, choose red or black but not refried, since they are high in fat. Avoid the rice. If a salad is available, enjoy a large one before your entrée.

Asian restaurants

These are usually good choices, provided your meat or seafood is baked, steamed, poached, or stir-fried. Steaming is usually the healthiest method. Instead of fried rice or fried noodles, choose brown rice. If permitted, substitute a serving of rice with vegetables. If that is not possible, don't eat more than a tennis-ball-sized serving of rice. Avoid sweet and sour, batter-fried, or twice-cooked food (which is high in fat and calories) and oily sauces (i.e., duck). For an appetizer you can choose wonton or egg drop soup instead of deep-fried egg rolls. Sushi is fine; some restaurants prepare it with brown rice.

Look for restaurants that do not use MSG or that will not use it on your dish. MSG has numerous potential reactions. The most common is stimulating your appetite, causing you to become hungry again in a couple hours. More importantly, MSG can lead to severe headaches, heart palpitations, and shortness of breath. (For more information on MSG, refer to my book *The Seven Pillars of Health*.)

Indian restaurants

Many Indian foods contain large portions of ghee (clarified butter) or oil, so it's best to find a restaurant willing to limit the amount they use on your dish. Tandoori-cooked (roasted) or grilled fish, chicken, beef, and shrimp are good choices. Avoid deep-fried foods and sauces, such as marsala sauce and curry sauce, which are high in fat. If you must have them, get them in a small side dish. Also, it's best to avoid the breads—a major element of Indian food. If you have any, however, choose bread that is baked (*nan*) instead of the fried *chapatis* bread.

Family-style restaurants

Foods at these restaurants are typically high in fats; the main courses are often fried. The vegetables are usually loaded with gravy, butter, or oil. Good choices include baked or grilled chicken, turkey, or beef with steamed vegetables. Vegetable or bean or lentil soup and a salad (dressing on the side) also make good choices. Avoid the large dinner rolls, butter, and fried side dishes. Choose beans, such as lima, pinto, or string beans. If you must have gravy, get it on the side and eat it sparingly. Though raised on Southern cooking, I have learned I can enjoy the foods without all the gravies and fried options.

> The LORD is my strength and my shield; my heart trusted in Him, and I am helped; therefore my heart greatly rejoices, and with my song I will praise Him.
> —PSALM 28:7

A FINAL WORD

Eating healthily is not a diet but a lifestyle. So follow this lifestyle every day. There will be times that you will slip, especially on holidays, birthdays, anniversaries, weddings, and other special occasions. However, never give up. Simply get back on the program, and you will again start burning fat and building muscle.

If you reach a plateau or if you are unable to lose more weight, simply avoid high-glycemic carbohydrates, which include breads, pasta, potatoes, corn, rice, pretzels, bagels, crackers, cereals, popcorn, beans, bananas, and dried fruit. Choose low-glycemic vegetables and fruits. If after a month or two of doing this you are still unable to lose sufficient weight, you should choose low-glycemic vegetables and salads and avoid fruits for approximately a month until you break through the plateau. Then reintroduce low-glycemic fruits.

I am praying for God to give you the determination and will power to follow through on this eating strategy. Not only will you lose weight, but also you will keep it off. In doing so, you will take care of your body, God's temple, and live a full and abundant life to His glory. Eat right and live in divine health!

A **BIBLE CURE** Prayer for You

Lord, You are my strength. I trust You to help me make healthy choices to reach and maintain a healthy weight even when I am away from home or celebrating with friends and family. I can cry out to You when I am tempted, and You will be there to help me. You never give me more than I can bear. I declare that I will walk in discipline and stay focused on maintaining a healthy lifestyle. In Jesus's name, amen.

A **BIBLE CURE** Prescription

Check the healthy choices you are willing to make when you are eating out:

❑ Plan ahead.

❑ Eat a snack beforehand and/or take PGX fiber supplements.

❑ Take half of my entrée to go.

❑ Avoid dessert.

❑ Other: _____

Write a prayer asking God for help in making wise choices when eating out:

_____

_____

_____

_____

Chapter 5

POWER FOR CHANGE THROUGH ACTIVITY

G OD HAS MADE you the master of your body—it is not the master of you! Too many of us let our bodies tell us what to do. However, God created this incredible body to be your servant. The apostle Paul revealed his understanding of this truth when he said, "I discipline my body and bring it into subjection, lest, when I have preached to others, I myself should become disqualified" (1 Cor. 9:27).

God has given you the power of mastery over your body. If you've let it get out of shape, it's time to assert your power!

> And let us not grow weary while doing good, for in due season we shall reap if we do not lose heart.
> —GALATIANS 6:9

Proper nutrition alone cannot reduce your weight sufficiently or adequately maintain your proper weight. However, proper nutrition combined with exercise will help you reach your goal of walking in divine health and living a long, wholesome life.

GET MOVING

There is no better way to complement a weight-loss dietary and supplement program than physical activity. It helps raise the metabolic rate during and after the activity. It enables you to develop more muscle, which raises the metabolic rate all day—even while you sleep. It decreases body fat and improves your ability to cope with stress by lowering the stress hormone cortisol.

Such activity also raises serotonin levels, which helps reduce cravings for sweets and carbohydrates. It assists in burning off dangerous belly fat and improves your body's ability to handle sugar. Finally, regular physical activity can even help control your appetite by boosting serotonin levels, lowering cortisol, and decreasing insulin levels (which can also decrease your chances for insulin resistance). Simply put, regular activity is extremely important if you want to lose weight and keep it off.

It's important to see your personal physician before starting a rigorous exercise program. Even if you have health considerations, you may be surprised to learn there are ways for you to become more active. Cycling, swimming, dancing, hiking, and sports such as basketball, volleyball, soccer, and tennis are all considered aerobic. Washing the car by hand, working in your yard, and mowing the grass qualify too. An aerobic exercise is simply something that uses large muscle groups of the body and raises the heart rate to a range that will burn fat for fuel. This is why aerobic exercise is one of the best ways to lose body fat.

A **BIBLE CURE** *Health Tip*
The Perks of Regular Activity

In case you needed a reminder, here are some of the many benefits that regular activity promotes:

- It decreases the risk of heart disease, stroke, and the development of hypertension.
- It helps prevent type 2 diabetes.
- It helps protect you from developing certain types of cancer.
- It helps prevent osteoporosis and aids in maintaining healthy bones.
- It helps prevent arthritis and aids in maintaining healthy joints.
- It slows down the overall aging process.
- It improves your mood and reduces the symptoms of anxiety and depression.
- It increases energy and mental alertness.
- It improves digestion.
- It gives you more restful sleep.
- It helps prevent colds and flu.
- It alleviates pain.
- It promotes weight loss and decreases appetite.

Try brisk walking. Brisk walking is the simplest and most convenient way to exercise aerobically. Walk briskly enough so that you can't sing, yet slow enough so that you can talk. This is a simple way to ensure you are entering your target heart rate zone. Diabetic patients with foot ulcers or numbness in the feet may want to avoid walking and should try cycling, an elliptical machine, or pool activities while inspecting the feet before and after activity.

Aerobic exercise will make you feel better immediately by putting more oxygen into your body. It also tones the heart and blood vessels, increases circulation, boosts the metabolic rate, improves digestion and elimination, controls insulin production, stimulates the production of neurotransmitters in the brain, improves the appetite and stimulates the lymphatic system, which aids in the removal of toxic material from the body.

Whatever activity you choose, the important thing is that you get moving regularly. Don't give yourself an excuse to justify a lack of activity. As you look for ways to increase your activity level, keep these tips in mind:

- Choose something that is fun and enjoyable. You will never stick to any activity program if you dread or hate it.

- Wear comfortable, well-fitting shoes and socks.

- If you are a type 1 diabetic, you will need to work with your doctor in order to adjust insulin doses while increasing your activity. Realize that exercising will lower your blood sugar; this can be potentially dangerous in a type 1 diabetic.

- The Centers for Disease Control and Prevention recommends brisk walking five days a week for thirty minutes. Start by walking only ten minutes a day and gradually increase your time to thirty minutes.

RECOMMENDED LEVEL OF INTENSITY

Every activity either requires or can be performed at different levels of intensity. Given that, it makes sense that every person hoping to lose weight has an ideal intensity at which he or she should work out. This is called your target heart rate zone, which generally ranges from 65 to 85 percent of your maximum heart rate.

To calculate the low end of this zone, start by subtracting your age from 220. This is your maximum heart rate. For example, for someone forty years old the formula is:

220 – 40 = 180 beats per minute

Multiply this number by 65 percent to find the low end of the target heart rate zone:

180 x 0.65 = 117 beats per minute

To figure out the high end of the zone, multiply maximum heart rate by 85 percent:

180 x 0.85 = 153 beats per minute

So, if you are forty, you should keep your heart rate between 117 and 153 beats per minute when exercising.

High-intensity aerobic exercise actually decreases insulin levels and increases levels of glucagon. By lowering insulin levels, you begin to release more stored body fat, and thus you burn fat, not carbohydrates. I recommend that you maintain a moderate pace as you exercise to keep your body burning fat as fuel.

When you exercise to the point that you are severely short of breath, you are no longer performing aerobically. Instead you have shifted to an anaerobic activity, which burns glycogen—stored sugar—as primary fuel instead of fat. I will explain the benefits of anaerobic activity a little later in this chapter. If you are just starting to exercise and aim to burn primarily fat, you need to work out at a moderate intensity of 65 to 85 percent of your maximum heart rate. This is the fat-burning range of your target heart rate zone.

When you start any activity program, I recommend you work out at around 65 percent of your maximum heart rate. As you become more aerobically conditioned, gradually increase the intensity to 70 percent of maximum heart rate. After a few more weeks, increase to 75 percent, and so on. You may never be able to work out at 85 percent of maximum rate, especially if you are huffing and puffing. Be sure that as you increase the intensity of your workouts, you remain able to converse with another person.

MUSCLES AND METABOLISM

Have you thought that having a high metabolism was others' blessing but not yours? It can be. Your metabolic rate is dependent upon your muscle mass. The more muscle mass you have, the higher your metabolic rate. If your dieting efforts do not include exercise, you can begin to burn muscle mass to supply your body with amino acids and sabotage your weight-loss efforts by slowing down your metabolic rate. The body will then begin to burn fewer calories and less fat. The more muscle you carry, the higher the metabolic rate and the more stored body fat you will burn—even at rest.

THE BENEFITS OF ANAEROBIC EXERCISE

Anaerobic exercise such as weightlifting, sprinting, and resistance training will help to increase lean muscle mass—thereby increasing your metabolic rate. If the workout is intense enough, growth hormone will be released from the pituitary gland. This leads to increased muscle growth and increased fat loss.

For maximum results, however, the exercise must be very strenuous and done until muscle exhaustion occurs or until you simply cannot move any more. This stimulates the release of a powerful surge of growth hormone, which helps to repair and rebuild the muscles that have been broken down during the workout. As you gain more muscle mass, your metabolic rate rises.

A word of caution, however: if you weigh yourself, the scale may not show a dramatic weight loss since the muscle mass that you are adding actually weighs more than the fat it is replacing.

I encourage my patients not to begin resistance training until they are in the routine of walking approximately thirty minutes five days a week. If you are just beginning a weight-lifting program, I recommend that you consult a certified personal trainer who will develop a well-rounded weight-lifting program for you.

As you exercise, be sure to maintain proper form and lift the weights slowly to avoid injury. You should typically perform ten to twelve repetitions per set. When starting resistance training, I recommend only performing one set per activity to reduce soreness. As you become better conditioned over time, you can increase to two or three sets per activity.

Increased sugar and increased starch will inhibit growth hormone release and is counterproductive. Therefore, prior to a workout, avoid snacks that are high in sugar or carbohydrates since you will not have the advantage of this powerful hormone for fat loss and muscle gain.

> He restores my soul; He leads me in the paths of righteousness for His name's sake.
> —PSALM 23:3

High-intensity interval training (HIIT) can also be an effective anaerobic workout. HIIT is simply alternating between brief, hard bursts of exercise and short stretches of lower-intensity exercise or rest, usually for a period of less than twenty minutes. Various studies in recent years have proven this to be an effective way to improve not only overall cardiovascular health but also your ability to burn fat faster. One study at the University of Guelph in Ontario, Canada, found that following an interval training session with an hour of moderate cycling increased the amount of fat burned by 36 percent.[1]

I personally do HIIT three times a week. I warm up on the elliptical machine for five to ten minutes. I then do sixty seconds of high-intensity training with high resistance and as fast as I can. I then decrease the resistance and speed to a lower setting for one minute. I continue this pattern for twenty minutes or more.

High-intensity anaerobic workouts obviously have proven value. However, I suggest that you hold off on HIIT, regardless of your exercise past, until you've consistently done some moderate-intensity activity for several months. I'd rather see you be able to sustain your momentum for the long haul rather than have you burn out, not because of eating the wrong things, but simply because you wanted to sprint to the finish line faster.

Be sure to have a physical exam with EKG and or a stress test before starting HIIT.

A **BIBLE CURE** Health Tip
The Tabata Method

A popular new form of HIIT is Tabata, an exercise regimen created by Izumi Tabata that uses twenty seconds of high-intensity exercise followed by ten seconds of rest, repeated for eight cycles. An alternative routine uses three minutes of warming up, followed by sixty seconds of high-intensity exercise, followed by seventy-five seconds of rest, repeated for eight to twelve cycles.

HOW MUCH EXERCISE IS ENOUGH?

The Centers for Disease Control and Prevention (CDC) and the National Institutes of Health (NIH) recommend that adults need two types of physical activity each week—aerobic and muscle-strengthening. For aerobic activity they recommend two hours and thirty minutes of moderate intensity aerobic activity (brisk walking, water aerobics, riding a bike on level ground, playing doubles tennis, pushing a lawn mower, etc.) every week, or one hour and fifteen minutes of vigorous exercise (jogging, swimming laps, riding a bike fast or on hills/inclines, playing singles tennis, playing basketball, etc.) every week. For muscle-strengthening exercise, which I call resistance exercise, they recommend two or more days a week, working all major muscle groups (legs, hips, back, abdomen, chest, shoulders, and arms).[2]

I recommend breaking up the aerobic activity as follows: if you can only do moderate intensity activities, try brisk walking for thirty minutes a day, five days a week. If you can handle more vigorous activity, jog for twenty-five minutes a day, three days a week. Or you can break it down even further: try going for a ten-minute walk, three times a day, five days a week.

MONITOR YOURSELF

I believe in monitoring yourself. An excellent way to monitor the steps you walk during the day is by using a pedometer. Typically a person walks three thousand to five thousand steps a day. To stay fit, set a goal of ten thousand steps, or approximately five miles. To lose weight, aim for between twelve thousand and fifteen thousand steps per day.

Before engaging in any activity, make sure that you have either eaten a meal two or three hours prior or have had a healthy snack about thirty to sixty minutes beforehand. It is never good to work out when hungry; you may end up burning muscle protein as energy—which is very expensive fuel. Remember, losing muscle lowers your metabolic rate.

> For He satisfies the longing soul, and fills the hungry soul with goodness.
>
> —PSALM 107:9

THE IMPORTANCE OF SLEEP

Another way to stimulate release of growth hormone to build muscle is to get a good night's sleep. Growth hormone is secreted during stage three and stage four sleep, which occur during the first couple of hours after falling asleep.

HITTING A PLATEAU

If you lose weight steadily and then seem to hit a plateau, exercise will help. By increasing the frequency and duration of exercise, you can break through that plateau and continue losing weight. Try to increase your exercise time gradually from thirty minutes to forty-five minutes. Those stubborn last few pounds will soon begin to melt away.

STEWARDING THE GIFT OF YOUR BODY

Your body is a wonderful gift. With God's help you can get into shape, feel better, and look fabulous. Determine right now to put these exercise tips into practice and, most importantly, to stay with it. Remember, everyone falls down, but it takes an individual with courage to get back up again. You will have your ups and downs—we all do. But hang in there. Stay with it. Before long you'll look like the person you've always dreamed of becoming!

A BIBLE CURE *Prayer for You*

Lord, I surrender all my cares to You. Give me the power of a disciplined life. Thank You for the gift of my body. I realize that it is a temple of the Holy Spirit and I must be a good steward of it. Each time I become discouraged or want to quit, please be there to pick me up and put me back on track. I surrender the care of my body to You and Your wonderful wisdom. In the name of Jesus Christ, amen.

A **BIBLE CURE** *Prescription*

Check the lifestyle changes you are willing to make to achieve weight loss:

❑ Exercise regularly. The type of exercise you will choose is:

_____

_____

❑ Get enough sleep.

❑ Begin a strengthening program.

❑ Other: _____

Write a prayer asking God for help in making these lifestyle changes.

_____

_____

_____

Write a prayer of commitment asking God for His help in staying faithful to an exercise program. Also, ask your spouse or a friend to exercise with you. An accountability partner increases the success of any weight loss program.

_____

_____

_____

Chapter 6

SUPPLEMENTS THAT SUPPORT WEIGHT LOSS

Your body is the temple of God's Spirit. The apostle Paul writes, "Do you not know that your body is the temple of the Holy Spirit who is in you, whom you have from God, and you are not your own? For you were bought at a price; therefore glorify God in your body and in your spirit, which are God's" (1 Cor. 6:19–20).

Your body is also the most incredible creation in the entire universe. All the money in the world could not replace it. It's God's awesome gift and a suitable place to house His own Spirit. Since your body was created as the temple of God's Spirit, it's important to understand that you and I are merely stewards of this gift God has given us.

If you went out today and purchased a Mercedes-Benz or a Porsche, no doubt you would polish it and fill it with the best gas and the best oil—treating it with the respect that such a fine machine deserves. You can honor God in your body as well by treating it with the respect and care that befits such a wonderful gift.

By giving your body the nutrients, vitamins, and minerals it needs to function at peak performance, you will bring honor to

God by properly caring for your body—the temple He created on earth to house His own Spirit.

WHAT IS YOUR BODY TRYING TO TELL YOU?

Your incredible body is so sophisticated that it is programmed to signal you that it needs a nutrient or a vitamin you haven't supplied. These signals come in the form of cravings. Have you ever just had to have a glass of orange juice? Your body was probably telling your brain that it needed more vitamin C.

> But those who wait on the LORD shall renew their strength; they shall mount up with wings like eagles, they shall run and not be weary, they shall walk and not faint.
>
> —ISAIAH 40:31

Cravings can come following a meal when the body realizes that, although it's been fed, it still hasn't received enough of the nutrients it expected. Too often, instead of discerning the craving properly, we simply fuel our bodies with even more non-nutritious food. Therefore the cravings return, and we respond once again with more junk food. The cycle becomes vicious, we get fatter, and our bodies suffer for lack of real nutrition.

If you experience such cravings, it's likely your body is actually slightly malnourished. Vitamins, minerals, and supplements are vital in today's world for the proper fueling of our bodies. You see, most old-time farmers know that in order for soil to supply the food it produces with a rich supply of vitamins and minerals, it must rest or lie fallow. In other words, it must remain unused every few years. In today's world of high-tech agriculture, this no longer occurs. Therefore our food supplies are actually depleted of the vitamins, minerals, and nutrients our bodies need to maintain good health. So we give our bodies more and more food, but they still lack vitamins and nutrients. That's where supplementation can bridge the gap.

NATURAL SUBSTANCES FOR YOU

Let's explore some of these natural substances that can promote health and vitality as you defeat obesity in your life. Since there are many causes of obesity, I recommend safe nutritional supplements that work through different mechanisms, such as thermogenic agents, natural appetite suppressants that increase satiety, supplements that increase insulin sensitivity, and energy products. We will also look at some of the supplements available that you should avoid as you take the necessary steps to reach your ideal weight.

Vitamins and minerals

A good multivitamin and multimineral. It's important to be sure that you get a good supply of all the various vitamins your body needs, especially if it is depleted. Most multivitamins contain only twelve vitamins in their inactive form. You may want to choose a multivitamin you can take two to three times a day. To prevent our adrenal glands from becoming exhausted, we need to supplement our diets daily with a comprehensive multivitamin and mineral formula with adequate amounts of B-complex vitamins. Divine Health Active Multivitamin has the active form of the vitamins, chelated minerals, and antioxidants in a balanced comprehensive formula.

Choosing a mineral supplement is a little more difficult than choosing a vitamin supplement and sometimes more costly. Find a mineral supplement that is chelated rather than one that contains mineral salts. Chelation is a process of wrapping a mineral with an organic molecule such as an amino acid that increases absorption dramatically. (See Appendix B.)

Green Supreme Food. This supplement contains fifteen organic fruits, veggies, and superfoods, as well as probiotics, fiber, antioxidants, and phytonutrients. It helps energize, detoxify, and create an alkaline environment in the tissue, helping one lose weight.

Thermogenic (fat-burning) agents

The term *thermogenic* describes the body's natural means of raising its temperature to burn off more calories. More specifically, thermogenesis is the process of triggering the body to burn white body fat, which is the kind of fat we often accumulate as we age. Thermogenic agents, then, are fat burners that help to increase the rate of white-body-fat breakdown. Fortunately, most unsafe thermogenic agents have been pulled off the market.

Green tea. Green tea and green tea extract are good weight-loss supplements. Green tea has been used for thousands of years in Asia as both a tea and an herbal medicine. It has two key ingredients: a catechin called epigallocatechin gallate (EGCG) and caffeine. Both lead to the release of more epinephrine, which then increases the metabolic rate. Ultimately green tea promotes fat oxidation, which is fat burning. It also increases the rate at which you burn calories over a twenty-four-hour period.

An effective daily dose of EGCG is 90 milligrams or more, which can be consumed by drinking three or four cups of green tea a day. Do not add sugar, honey, or artificial sweeteners to it, though you may use the natural sweetener stevia. In addition to drinking green tea, I recommend 100 milligrams of green tea supplement three times a day. (See Appendix B.)

> It is vain for you to rise up early, to sit up late, to eat the bread of sorrows; for so He gives His beloved sleep.
> —Psalm 127:2

Green coffee bean extract. A placebo-controlled study reported in January 2012 that green coffee bean extract produced weight loss in 100 percent of overweight participants. For twenty-two weeks participants were given 350 milligrams of green coffee bean extract twice a day. They did not change their diets, averaging 2,400 calories per day, but they did burn 400 calories a day through exercise. The average weight loss was 17.6 pounds, with some subjects losing 22.7 pounds, and there were no side effects.[1]

The key phytonutrient in green coffee bean extract is chlorogenic acid, which has the ability to decrease the uptake of glucose, fats, and carbohydrates from the intestines and thus decrease the absorption of calories. It also has positive effects on how your body processes glucose and fats, and it helps to lower blood sugar and insulin levels. Drinking coffee doesn't give you the same effects. Because of roasting, most of the chlorogenic acid in coffee is destroyed. By comparison, the extract is much better. Green coffee bean extract should contain 45 percent or more of chlorogenic acid. In addition to—or in place of—drinking coffee, I recommend taking 400 milligrams of green coffee bean extract thirty minutes before each meal. (See Appendix B.)

Meratrim. Meratrim is a blend of two plant extracts that has been shown to significantly reduce body weight, BMI, and waist measurement within eight weeks when used with a diet and exercise plan. The studies show that 400 milligrams of Meratrim twice a day, thirty minutes before breakfast and thirty minutes before dinner, achieved these results by interfering with the accumulation of fat while simultaneously increasing fat burning.[2] (See Appendix B.)

Thyroid support

All obese patients should be screened for hypothyroidism, using tests such as the blood tests TSH, free T3, free T4, and thyroid peroxidase antibodies, to rule out Hashimoto's thyroiditis, the most common cause of low thyroid. If a patient has low body temperature (less than 98 degrees), they most likely have a sluggish metabolism and may have sluggish thyroid function. It's especially important to optimize the free T3 blood level to improve the metabolic rate. The normal range of T3, according to the lab I use, is 2.1 to 4.4. I try to optimize the T3 level to a range of 3.0 to 4.2 by using both levothyroxine (T4) and liothyronine (T3). I can sometimes optimize the T3 levels with natural supplements including Metabolic Advantage or iodine supplements. I also commonly perform a lab test to see if a patient is low in iodine before starting iodine supplements. According to the American Thyroid Association, 40 percent of the world's population is at risk for iodine deficiency.[3]

Appetite suppressants

These supplements generally act on the central nervous system to decrease appetite or create a sensation of fullness. Although some medications in this category include risk-prone phenylpropanolamine (found in such products as Dexatrim), I have found a few safe, natural supplements that are extremely effective appetite suppressants.

L-tryptophan and 5-HTP. These are amino acids that help the body to manufacture serotonin. Serotonin assists in controlling carbohydrate and sugar cravings. L-tryptophan and 5-HTP also function like natural antidepressants. If you are taking migraine medications called triptans or SSRIs (selective serotonin reuptake inhibitors), you should talk with your physician before taking either supplement. The typical dose of L-tryptophan is 500 to 2,000 milligrams at bedtime. For 5-HTP it is typically 50 to 100 milligrams one to three times a day or 100 to 300 milligrams at bedtime. Serotonin Max is an excellent supplement that helps boost serotonin levels naturally. (See Appendix B.)

L-tyrosine, N-acetyl L-tyrosine, and L-phenylalanine. These are naturally occurring amino acids found in numerous protein foods, including cottage cheese, turkey, and chicken. They help to raise norepinephrine and dopamine levels in the brain, which then helps decrease appetite and cravings and improves your mood. Doses of L-tyrosine, N-acetyl L-tyrosine, and L-phenylalanine may range from 500 to 2,000 milligrams a day (sometimes higher), but they should be taken on an empty stomach. I prefer N-acetyl L-tyrosine for most of my patients since the body absorbs it better than L-tyrosine or L-phenylalanine. I typically start patients on 500 to 1,000 milligrams of N-acetyl L-tyrosine, taken thirty minutes before breakfast and thirty minutes before lunch. I do not recommend taking any of these supplements in late afternoon because they may interfere with sleep. (See Appendix B.)

Supplements to increase satiety

Fiber supplements and foods high in fiber increase feelings of fullness by using several different mechanisms. Fiber slows the passage of food through the digestive tract, decreases the absorption of sugars and starches into the stomach, and expands and fills up the stomach—turning down the appetite. Although the American Heart Association and the National Cancer Institute recommend 30 grams or more of fiber each day, the average American only consumes between 12 and 17 grams.[4]

When it comes to losing weight and managing blood sugar levels, a little fiber goes a long way. One study found that consuming an extra 14 grams of soluble fiber each day for only two days was associated with a 10 percent decrease in caloric intake.[5] Soluble fiber supplements significantly increase post-meal satisfaction and should be taken before each meal to assist in weight loss. Soluble fiber lowers the blood sugar, slowing down digestion and the absorption of sugars and carbohydrates. This allows for a more gradual rise in blood sugar, which lowers the glycemic index of the foods you eat. This helps to improve the blood sugar levels.

The fiber that I prefer for weight-loss patients is PGX. I start with one capsule, taken with 8 to 16 ounces of water before each meal and snack, and then gradually increase the dose to two to four capsules until patients can control their appetite. Always take PGX with evening meals and snacks.

In addition to PGX, another great fiber for weight loss is glucomannan, made from the Asian root konjac. Glucomannan is five times more effective in lowering cholesterol when compared to other fibers such as psyllium, oat fiber, or guar gum. Because it expands to ten times its original size when placed in water, it is a great supplement to take before a meal to reduce your appetite as it expands in your stomach, but you should take it with 16 ounces of water or unsweetened black or green tea. (See Appendix B.)

Supplements to increase energy production

L-carnitine is an amino acid that helps our bodies turn food into energy by shuttling fatty acids into the mitochondria, which act as our cells' energy factories by burning fatty acids for energy. Humans synthesize very little carnitine, so we may need to supplement from outside sources. This applies especially to obese and older individuals, who typically have lower levels of carnitine than the average-weight segment of the population. As you might expect, individuals with insufficient carnitine have a greater difficulty burning fat for energy.

> For the kingdom of God is not eating and drinking, but righteousness and peace and joy in the Holy Spirit.
> —ROMANS 14:17

Milk, meat such as mutton and lamb, fish, and cheese are good sources of L-carnitine. In supplement form, I recommend taking a combination of L-carnitine and acetyl-L-carnitine, lipoic acid, PQQ (pyrroloquinoline quinone), and a glutathione-boosting supplement. The best time to take these supplements is in the morning and early afternoon (before 3:00 p.m.) on an empty stomach. If you take them any later, these supplements can impair your sleep. Green tea supplements and N-acetyl L-tyrosine also help to increase your energy.

Other common supplements to assist with weight loss

Irvingia. Irvingia is a fruit-bearing plant grown in the jungles of Cameroon in Africa. Irvingia gabonensis helps to resensitize your cells to insulin. It appears to be able to reverse leptin resistance by lowering levels of C-reactive protein (CRP), an inflammatory mediator. Leptin is a hormone that tells your brain you've eaten enough and that it is time to stop. It also enhances your body's ability to use fat as an energy source. One also needs zinc, 12 to 15 milligrams a day, which is present in most comprehensive multivitamins, in order for leptin to function optimally.

Because of Americans' sedentary lifestyles and highly processed, high-glycemic food choices, many overweight and obese patients have acquired resistance to leptin. As a result, this hormone no longer works properly in their bodies. Similar to insulin resistance, leptin resistance is a chronic inflammatory condition that contributes to weight gain. It is critically important to follow the anti-inflammatory dietary program I have outlined in this book. Simply decreasing inflammatory foods enables most to start losing belly fat and also allows leptin to function optimally. The generally recommended dose is 150 milligrams of standardized Irvingia extract, twice a day, thirty minutes before lunch and dinner.

7-keto-DHEA. Derived from the hormone dehydroepiandrosterone (DHEA), 7-keto-DHEA is taken to help rev a person's metabolism to aid in weight loss. Unlike its "parent hormone" DHEA, which is produced by glands near the kidneys, 7-keto-DHEA does not affect sex hormone levels in the body.[6] The supplement is also used to improve lean body mass, build muscle, boost the immune system, enhance memory, and slow aging, though there is limited scientific evidence to support all of those benefits.[7] However, 7-keto-DHEA has been shown to increase the resting metabolic rate in those who were already dieting and engaging in regular exercise. An eight-week study found that those who took 100 mg of 7-keto-DHEA twice a day lost about six pounds while those who received a placebo lost a little over two pounds.[8] The supplement was not found to have any adverse side effects after a series of toxicological evaluations. A safety study published in *Clinical Investigative Medicine* indicated that 7-keto-DHEA was safe for human consumption in doses of 200 mg per day for up to four weeks. The safety of internal use beyond four weeks is not known.[9]

The hoodia controversy. Hoodia is a South African plant similar to a cactus that may help suppress the appetite. Initially used by tribal leaders to enable them to go on long journeys without getting hungry, various sources cite thousands of years' worth of Bushman history to verify its effectiveness. Although these tribal hunters obviously have not conducted scientific studies to prove hoodia is an effective appetite suppressant, one 2001 clinical study by a company called Phytopharm found individuals who consumed the plant ate 1,000 fewer calories a day than those who didn't take hoodia.[10] One of the company's researchers, Richard Dixey, MD, explained that hoodia contains a molecule that is ten thousand times more active than glucose.[11] However, there is a catch. When news of this supposed miracle supplement hit the headlines, dozens (if not hundreds) of companies started marketing hoodia—without having any actual hoodia in their products. The result was that more hoodia was "produced" in a single year than in all of African history—highly unlikely, to say the least. Even today it is possible that much of what is sold in the United States either contains ineffective hoodia variations or no hoodia. So be wary of falling for marketing schemes with this substance.

NO MAGIC BULLET

There is no magic weight-loss pill. Scientists have been searching for "The Pill to End All Diets" for years, and no magic bullet has been found. There have been several attempts, including the popular fen-phen back in the nineties. While individuals lost weight, after only a few years a small percentage of users died of a rare disease called primary pulmonary hypertension. This affected several patients out of one hundred thousand; about half of them eventually required a heart-lung transplant to survive. The drug was eventually pulled, and several years later another miracle cure seemed to emerge. Combining ephedra with caffeine seemed to be a powerful formula for turning down the appetite and burning fat. But in time the safety of ephedra was also called into question. It has been linked with severe side effects, including arrhythmias, heart attack, stroke, hypertension, psychosis, seizure, and even death.

Due to safety concerns, in 2004 the Food and Drug Administration (FDA) banned ephedra products in the United States. Although a federal court later upheld the ban, companies wiggle around it by selling extracts that contain little or no ephedrine. And some related herbs, such as bitter orange (citrus aurantium) and country mallow, remain on the market. Like ephedra, bitter orange supplements have been linked to stroke, cardiac arrest, angina, heart attack, ventricular arrhythmias, and death. These products are potentially lethal. I do not recommend them unless taken under the direction and close monitoring of a knowledgeable physician.

A **BIBLE CURE** *Health Fact*
Alli and Hydroxycut Side Effects

Alli, one of the most common over-the-counter diet pills, may cause bowel changes in its users. These changes, which result from undigested fat going through the digestive system, may include gas with an oily discharge, loose stools or diarrhea, more frequent and urgent bowel movements, and hard-to-control bowel movements. Hydroxycut products were recalled in May 2009 after reports of deadly liver failure and disease in individuals who took the products to lose weight. According to the *World Journal of Gastroenterology*, an ingredient in Hydroxycut from a fruit called Garcinia cambogia caused the liver disease and failure.[12]

Among other herbs of concern is aristolochia, which is found in some Chinese herbal weight-loss supplements and may not even be listed as an ingredient. Aristolochia is a known kidney toxin and carcinogen in humans. There are also products containing usnea (usnic acid), a lichen for weight loss that can cause severe liver toxicity. In addition, some Brazilian diet pills have been found to be contaminated with amphetamines and other prescription drugs.[13]

A weight-loss supplement is a nutritional product or herb intended to assist your healthy eating and activity plan with the ultimate goal of losing weight. A supplement comes alongside; it does not replace. Do not be deceived by crafty marketing that promises otherwise. Weight-loss and dietary supplements are not subject to the same standards as prescription drugs or medications sold over the counter. They can be marketed with only limited proof of safety or effectiveness.

> Therefore, if anyone is in Christ, he is a new creation; old things have passed away; behold, all things have become new.
> —2 CORINTHIANS 5:17

A LIFESTYLE CHOICE

While some questionable products are on the market, there are a variety of safe, effective over-the-counter dietary supplements for weight loss. Some people may find that incorporating a combination of these into their eating and activity plan works even better. Others may not need to take any supplements. Most of my overweight and obese patients have found that taking a combination of green tea extract, green coffee bean extract, and Irvingia (see Appendix B) along with certain amino acids (such as Serotonin Max and N-acetyl L-tyrosine), and PGX fiber supplements before each meal and snack (especially in the evening) helped them shed pounds and controlled their appetites. (See Appendix B.)

If you continue experiencing problems controlling your appetite or struggle with food cravings, decreased energy, or insulin resistance, you will likely require one or more of the supplements I just reviewed. The same goes if you do not feel full or satisfied after a meal or if you have low hormone levels.

However, I remind you that supplements are just that—supplements, not magic pills. The truth is that there is no shortcut to losing weight and keeping it off. A new lifestyle that includes good nutrition, exercise, supplementation, and constant diligence is the best way to overcome obesity. The vitamins and supplements I have suggested can help you, but only you can decide to begin an entirely new lifestyle filled with health, vitality, and God's very best! Make that determination at this very moment.

A **BIBLE CURE** *Prayer for You*

Lord, thank You for vitamins and supplements that can help me battle obesity. Help me to be diligent in a plan to overcome obesity and to live a healthy lifestyle guided by Your Spirit and plan for divine health. Amen.

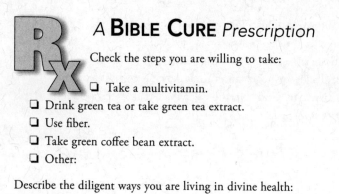

A BIBLE CURE Prescription

Check the steps you are willing to take:

❑ Take a multivitamin.

❑ Drink green tea or take green tea extract.

❑ Use fiber.

❑ Take green coffee bean extract.

❑ Other:

Describe the diligent ways you are living in divine health:

_____

_____

_____

_____

_____

_____

_____

_____

_____

Chapter 7

POWER FOR CHANGE THROUGH FAITH IN GOD

THERE IS NO greater love in the universe than the love God feels for you. No matter what you've done or neglected to do, He loves you more than you could ever know. And He longs to reveal His love to you in every place of emotional need. He tenderly calls you—even now—asking you to give Him all of the hurts, hidden pain, and disappointments that you've been carrying around with you. The Bible instructs us, "Casting all your care upon Him, for He cares about you" (1 Pet. 5:7).

Look at what Jesus said in Matthew 11:28: "Come to Me." How often have you—for lack of comfort, nervousness, because of a numb inability to really face your emotional pain, or from a hollow sense of aloneness—opened up the refrigerator and filled an empty place in your heart with a piece of pie or a cupcake?

You see, just as with a drug, food can temporarily anesthetize you from the pain of loneliness, abandonment, fear, stress, and emotional pain. It's no wonder the American population is getting larger. We are a nation emotionally hurting from a lack of love. But food cannot truly fill that void—even if we haven't faced it for so long that we hardly notice it anymore.

> Being confident of this very thing, that He who has begun a good work in you will complete it until the day of Jesus Christ.
>
> —PHILIPPIANS 1:6

But I have really good news for you. Jesus Christ can fill it, and He can comfort your heart with a sense of peace that will overwhelm you with true joy.

You see, Jesus Christ died for you in order to meet your need and comfort your pain. And He is just as alive today and as real as when He walked the shores of Galilee. Make the choice to let Him tenderly love you. All you need to do is ask Him. His love is just the whisper of a prayer away.

FEELING GUILTY ABOUT FOOD CRAVINGS?

Have you ever felt that your cravings for certain foods were somehow a guilty reflection upon you? Unhealthy food cravings are merely your body's way of signaling you that something is out of whack. From now on, commit your cravings to God at the moment they occur. He will give you the strength to get through them without overeating and the grace and wisdom to understand what your body or heart is trying to tell you. Let your cravings begin a process of bringing your body back into physical and spiritual balance, and with that balance, better health. One of the main emotional motivators that can send you racing to the refrigerator for comfort is stress. Stress works against you in other ways too.

STRESS CAN MAKE YOU FAT

The excessive stress you are under on a daily basis can contribute to obesity. When you are under stress, your body produces a hormone called cortisol, which is very similar to cortisone. If you have ever taken cortisone, you are well aware of the side effects. Cortisone causes you to gain weight.

Cortisol can have the same effect. When your adrenal glands produce cortisol during periods of high anxiety and stress, it can actually cause your body to gain weight. Therefore reducing your level of stress can help you lose weight and keep it off.

A CLOSER LOOK

Stress affects the heart, the blood vessels, and the immune system, but it also directly affects our adrenal glands. The adrenal glands, along with the thyroid gland, help to maintain the body's energy levels. God's plan for your life will help you to lower your stress. His plan for you is good and not bad. "For I know the thoughts that I think toward you, says the LORD, thoughts of peace and not of evil, to give you a future and a hope. Then you will call upon Me and go and pray to Me, and I will listen to you. And you will seek Me and find Me, when you search for Me with all your heart" (Jer. 29:11–13).

THE POWER OF SCRIPTURE

God wants you to surrender your cares to Him and allow His peace to rule in your heart. Memorize and meditate on these two promises for your life:

Be anxious for nothing, but in everything by prayer and supplication, with thanksgiving, let your requests be made known to God; and the peace of God, which surpasses all understanding, will guard your hearts and minds through Christ Jesus.

—PHILIPPIANS 4:6–7

Casting all your care upon Him, for He cares for you.

—1 PETER 5:7

When you hold on to your worries and cares, you find yourself under stress and overeating or not watching what you eat. When you are depressed and believing the worst is yet to come, you may try to use food as comfort. Trust God's Word and plan for your life, and turn all your cares and worries over to Him.

THE COMFORTER IS COME

God knows how tough our lives can be and how often we face life's difficulties alone. That's why He provided Himself as our Comforter. When the light goes on inside of your heart, when you really understand that God is real, that He is alive, that you are not alone, and that He is able to provide you the comfort you need, you will never reach for the empty comfort of food again. I encourage you to study the scriptures throughout this Bible Cure; read them over and over again. At the moment you are tempted to reach for comfort from food, read a verse and pray. God is able to give you the strength and help you need to overcome any and all emotional aspects of obesity. He will set you completely free.

THE BREAD OF LIFE

Jesus says that He is the bread of life. When you feel emotional cravings for sweets, carbohydrates, and other foods that you do not need, turn to the bread that you need—Jesus Christ. Let your cravings for rich food be transformed into signals that turn you to true riches in Christ. Remember His words:

> I am the bread of life. He who comes to Me shall never hunger, and he who believes in Me shall never thirst.
>
> —JOHN 6:35

As you've read through this book, I hope you've discovered that although God is very powerful, He came to share His power with you. You are not powerless in the face of temptation, fear, loneliness, or confusion. One of the most wonderful things about Jesus Christ is that He is very near. Reach out to Him for all of your needs. You will not be disappointed.

A BIBLE CURE Prayer for You

Lord God, You alone are my strength and my source. My ability to stay committed to weight loss and healthy eating comes from You. Help me maintain the willpower I need. Give me the focus I need to implement all that I am learning. Almighty God, replace any discouragement with hope and any doubt with faith. I know that You are with me and will not leave me. I thank You, Lord, for seeing me through this battle and giving me victory over obesity. Amen.

A **BIBLE CURE** *Prescription*

This is a daily checklist to copy and keep on your refrigerator, in your purse, or in your briefcase. Do each one daily for best results.

❏ I awakened and confessed that this body belongs to Jesus, and I'll give my body what it needs and not what it craves.

❏ I can do all things through Christ who strengthens me, and that includes losing weight.

❏ I thanked God throughout the day that I am slender and energetic, my health is restored, and my strength is renewed. (You may not be slender now, but start saying it by faith.)

❏ I ate a balanced breakfast, lunch, dinner, and snack according to the Bible Cure plan.

❏ I determined to walk in faith today with God's help.

❏ I took vitamins and supplements according to the Bible Cure plan. I exercised according to the Bible Cure plan.

❏ I feel strong and disciplined with God's help.

❏ I thank God throughout the day because now losing weight is easy for me.

A PERSONAL NOTE
From Don Colbert

GOD DESIRES TO heal you of disease. His Word is full of promises that confirm His love for you and His desire to give you His abundant life. His desire includes more than physical health for you; He wants to make you whole in your mind and spirit as well as through a personal relationship with His Son, Jesus Christ.

If you haven't met my best friend, Jesus, I would like to take this opportunity to introduce Him to you. It is very simple. If you are ready to let Him come into your life and become your best friend, all you need to do is sincerely pray this prayer:

> *Lord Jesus, I want to know You as my Savior and Lord. I believe You are the Son of God and that You died for my sins. I also believe You were raised from the dead and now sit at the right hand of the Father praying for me. I ask You to forgive me for my sins and change my heart so that I can be Your child and live with You eternally. Thank You for Your peace. Help me to walk with You so that I can begin to know You as my best friend and my Lord. Amen.*

If you have prayed this prayer, you have just made the most important decision of your life. I rejoice with you in your decision and your new relationship with Jesus. Please contact my publisher at pray4me@charismamedia.com so that we can send you some materials that will help you become established in your relationship with the Lord. We look forward to hearing from you.

Appendix A

THE BIBLE CURE'S SIMPLE RULES FOR WEIGHT LOSS

THE FOLLOWING ARE simple dieting rules that I always recommend to my patients who need to lose weight:

1. Graze throughout the day. (Eat lots of salads and veggies often throughout the day, and eat beans, peas, or lentils once or twice a day, up to four cups daily.)

2. Eat a large breakfast. Eat breakfast like a king, lunch like a prince, and dinner like a pauper. Eat smaller midmorning and midafternoon snacks.

3. Avoid all simple-sugar foods, i.e., candies, cookies, cakes, pies, and doughnuts. If you must have sugar, use either stevia, xylitol, Sweet Balance, Just Like Sugar (found in health food stores), or small amounts of coconut sugar or tagatose.

4. Drink two quarts of filtered or bottled water a day. That includes 16 ounces thirty minutes before each meal, or one to two 8-ounce glasses two and a half hours after each meal. Also, drink 8 to 16 ounces of water upon awakening.

5. Avoid alcohol and all fried foods.

6. For meals, choose a lean protein, a low-glycemic carb, and a healthy fat (but do your best to go "carb free" and low fat after 3:00 p.m.). Serving sizes for protein are typically 3 ounces for women and 3 to 6 ounces for men. Limit red meat intake to a maximum of 12 ounces per week.

7. Soups should be low-sodium and broth-based, not cream-based; vegetable, bean, pea, and lentil soups are good options. Use Himalayan or Celtic sea salt instead of regular table salt (less than 1 teaspoon a day).

8. If organic foods are too expensive, choose organic for the foods you consume most often. If you can't buy organic, then choose very lean cuts of meat, peel the skin off poultry, thoroughly wash fruits and vegetables that cannot be peeled, and choose skim milk or 1 percent dairy products and skim milk cheese.

9. Avoid high-glycemic starches, including wheat and corn products, or at least decrease them dramatically. This includes all breads, crackers, bagels, potatoes, pasta, white rice, and corn. Avoid bananas and dried fruit.

10. Eat fresh, low-glycemic fruits only for breakfast or lunch and occasionally with morning and early afternoon snacks; eat steamed, stir-fried, or raw vegetables, lean meats, salads with colorful vegetables (preferably with a salad spritzer), raw nuts, and seeds.

11. Take fiber supplements such as two to four capsules of PGX fiber with 16 ounces of water before each meal and two to three PGX fiber capsules with each snack.

12. Do not eat later than 7:00 p.m.

RESOURCES FOR WEIGHT LOSS

Most of the products mentioned throughout this book are offered through Dr. Colbert's Divine Health Wellness Center or are available at your local health food store.

Divine Health Nutritional Products
1908 Boothe Circle
Longwood, FL 32750
Phone: (407) 331-7007
Web site: www.drcolbert.com
E-mail: info@drcolbert.com

Maintenance nutritional supplements
- Divine Health Active Multivitamin
- Divine Health Living Multivitamin
- Divine Health Green Supreme Food

Omega oils
- Divine Health Living Omega

Protein powders
- Divine Health Plant Protein
- Divine Health Living Protein

Supplements for weight loss
- Fat Loss Drops

- PGX fiber
- Living Green Tea with EGCG
- Living Green Coffee Bean
- Meratrim (Metabolic Lean)
- MBS 360: contains green coffee bean and green tea with EGCG and Irvingia (available at www .mbs360.tv) This contains three fat-burners in one pill.
- 7-keto-DHEA

Supplements for thyroid support
- Metabolic Advantage
- Iodine Synergy

To curb food cravings
- Serotonin Max
- N-acetyl-tyrosine
- 5-HTP

Supplements to boost energy
- Divine Health Adrenal Support
- Divine Health PQQ
- Cellgevity (supplement to quench inflammation)

NOTES

INTRODUCTION
YOU ARE GOD'S MASTERPIECE!

1. Centers for Disease Control and Prevention (CDC), "Overweight and Obesity: Defining Overweight and Obesity," http://www.cdc.gov /obesity/adult/defining.html (accessed March 19, 2013).

2. Centers for Disease Control and Prevention (CDC), "FastStats: Obesity and Overweight," http://www.cdc.gov/nchs/fastats/overwt.htm (accessed March 19, 2013).

3. Department of Health and Human Services, "Overweight and Obesity: Health Consequences," http://www.surgeongeneral.gov/library /calls/obesity/fact_consequences.html (accessed March 7, 2013).

4. Eric A. Finkelstein, Justin G. Trogdon, Joel W. Cohen, and William Dietz, "Annual Medical Spending Attributable to Obesity: Payer- and Service-Specific Estimates," *Health Affairs* 28, no. 5 (July 27, 2009): w822-w831; http://content.healthaffairs.org/content/28/5/w822.full .pdf+html (accessed March 7, 2013).

CHAPTER 1
DID YOU KNOW?—UNDERSTANDING OBESITY

1. Alicia G. Walton, "How Much Sugar Are Americans Eating [Infographic]," Forbes.com, August 30, 2012, http://www.forbes.com/sites /alicegwalton/2012/08/30/how-much-sugar-are-americans-eating -infographic/ (accessed March 7, 2013).

2. William Davis, *Wheat Belly* (New York: Rodale, 2011), 14.

3. H. C. Broeck, H. C. de Jong, E. M. Salentijn, et al., "Presence of Celiac Disease Epitopes in Modern and Old Hexaploid Wheat Varieties: Wheat Breeding May Have Contributed to Increased Prevalence of Celiac Disease," *Theoretical and Applied Genetics* 121, no. 8 (November 2010): 1527–1539, as referenced in Davis, *Wheat Belly*, 26.

4. Davis, *Wheat Belly*, 35.

5. Ibid., 36. 53–54.

6. Ibid., 45.

7. Based on chart at BestDietTips.com, "Glycemic Index Food List (GI)," http://www.bestdiettips.com/glycemic-index-food-list-high-and-low-gi -index-foods-chart (accessed March 19, 2013).

8. Natalie Digate Muth, "Ask an Expert: What Are the Guidelines for Percentage of Body Fat Loss?" The American Council on Exercise, December 2, 2009, http://www.acefitness.org/acefit/expert-insight -article/3/112/what-are-the-guidelines-for-percentage-of/ (accessed May 2, 2013).

CHAPTER 2
THE FOUNDATION OF HEALTHY EATING

1. US Department of Health and Human Services, *Dietary Guidelines for Americans, 2010*, 7th ed. (Washington DC: US Government Printing Office, 2010), 15; viewed at http://health.gov/dietaryguidelines /dga2010/DietaryGuidelines2010.pdf (accessed March 20, 2013).
2. Kate Murphy, "The Dark Side of Soy," BusinessWeek.com, December 18, 2000, http://www.businessweek.com/2000/00_51/b3712218.htm (accessed September 17, 2009).

CHAPTER 3
POWER FOR CHANGE THROUGH DIET AND NUTRITION

1. MedicalNewsToday.com, "Mediterranean-Style Diet Reduces Cancer and Heart Disease Risk," June 26, 2003, http://www .medicalnewstoday.com/articles/3835.php (accessed March 20, 2013).
2. Antonia Trichopoulou, Pagona Lagiou, Hannah Kupeer, and Dimitrios Trichopoulos, "Cancer and the Mediterranean Dietary Traditions," *Cancer Epidemiology, Biomarkers and Prevention* 9 (September 2009): 869–873.
3. Gina Kolata, "Mediterranean Diet Shown to Ward Off Heart Attack and Stroke," *New York Times*, February 25, 2013, http://www.nytimes .com/2013/02/26/health/mediterranean-diet-can-cut-heart-disease -study-finds.html?pagewanted=all&_r=0 (accessed May 1, 2013).
4. Clara Felix, *All About Omega-3 Oils* (Garden City, NY: Avery Publishing, 1998), 32.
5. "Mercury Contamination in Fish: A Guide to Staying Healthy and Fighting Back," Natural Resources Defense Council, http://www .nrdc.org/health/effects/mercury/guide.asp (accessed May 1, 2013).

6. Robert Preidt, "Mom Was Right: Eating Soup Cuts Calorie Intake," May 1, 2007, ABCNews.com, http://abcnews.go.com/Health /Healthday/story?id=4506787&page=1 (accessed March 21, 2013).
7. Jennie Brand-Miller, Thomas M. S. Wolever, Kaye Foster-Powell, and Stephen Colagiuri, *The New Glucose Revolution*, 3rd ed., (New York: Marlow & Co., 2007), 86.
8. ScienceDaily.com, "Teens Who Eat Breakfast Daily Eat Healthier Diets Than Those Who Skip Breakfast," March 3, 2008, http://www .sciencedaily.com/releases/2008/03/080303072640.htm (accessed March 21, 2013).
9. K. N. Boutelle and D. S. Kirschenbaum, "Further Support for Consistent Self-Monitoring as a Vital Component of Successful Weight Control," *Obesity Research* 6, no. 3 (May 1998): 219–224, http:// www.ncbi.nlm.nih.gov/pubmed/9618126 (accessed March 21, 2013).

CHAPTER 4
TIPS FOR EATING OUT

1. National Restaurant Association, "Restaurant Industry Sales Turn Positive in 2011 After Three Tough Years," RestaurantNews.com, February 1, 2011, http://www.restaurantnews.com/restaurant-industry -sales-turn-positive-in-2011-after-three-tough-years/ (accessed March 26, 2013).

CHAPTER 5
POWER FOR CHANGE THROUGH ACTIVITY

1. Peter Jaret, "A Healthy Mix of Rest and Motion," *New York Times*, May 3, 2007, http://tinyurl.com/c7zxot3 (accessed March 26, 2013).
2. Centers for Disease Control and Prevention, "How Much Physical Activity Do Adults Need?", December 1, 2011, http://www.cdc.gov /physicalactivity/everyone/guidelines/adults.html (accessed March 26, 2013).

CHAPTER 6
SUPPLEMENTS THAT SUPPORT WEIGHT LOSS

1. LifeExtension.org, "Journal Abstracts: Green Coffee Bean Extract," *Life Extension Magazine*, February 2012, http://www.lef.org/magazine/mag2012/abstracts/feb2012_Green-Coffee-Bean-Extract_04.htm (accessed March 26, 2013).

2. Douglas Laboratories, "Metabolic Lean: Weight Management Formula," product data sheet, June 2012, http://www.douglaslabs.com/pdf/pds/201350.pdf (accessed March 26, 2013).

3. American Thyroid Association, "Iodine Deficiency," June 4, 2012, http://www.thyroid.org/iodine-deficiency/ (accessed March 26, 2013).

4. J. A. Marlett, M. I. McBurney, J. L. Slavin, and American Dietetic Association, "Position of the American Dietetic Association: Health Implications of Dietary Fiber," *Journal of the American Dietetic Association* 102, no. 7 (2002): 993–1000.

5. N. C. Howarth, E. Saltzman, and S. B. Roberts, "Dietary Fiber and Weight Regulation," *Nutrition Review* 59, no. 5 (2001): 129–138.

6. Andrew Weil, "7-Keto: Supplement to Speed Metabolism?" DrWeil.com, http://www.drweil.com/drw/u/QAA401158/7Keto-Supplement-to-Speed-Metabolism.html (accessed May 2, 2013).

7. "7-Keto-DHEA," WebMD.com, http://www.webmd.com/vitamins-supplements/ingredientmono-835-7-KETO-DHEA.aspx?active IngredientId=835&activeIngredientName=7-KETO-DHEA (accessed May 2, 2013).

8. Weil, "7-Keto: Supplement to Speed Metabolism?"

9. J. L. Zenk, J. L. Frestedt, and M. A. Kuskowski, "HUM5007, a Novel Combination of Thermogenic Compounds, and 3-Acetyl-7-Oxo-Dehydroepiandrosterone: Each Increases the Resting Metabolic Rate of Overweight Adults," *Journal of Nutritional Biochemistry* 18, no. 9 (September 2007): 629–634; and Michael Davidson, Ashok Marwah, Ronald J. Sawchuk, et. al., "Safety and Pharmacokinetic Study With Escalating Doses of 3-Acetyl-7-Oxo-Dehydroepiandrosterone in Healthy Male volunteers," *Clinical Investigative Medicine* 23, no. 5 (October 2000): 300-310, abstract viewed at http://www.ncbi.nlm.nih.gov/pubmed/11055323 (accessed May 2, 2013).

10. Hoodia Advice, "The Science of Hoodia," http://www.hoodia-advice
    .org/hoodia-plant.html (accessed March 26, 2013).

11. Tom Mangold, "Sampling the Kalahari Hoodia Diet," BBC News,
    May 30, 2003, http://news.bbc.co.uk/2/hi/programmes
    /correspondent/2947810.stm (accessed March 26, 2013).

12. Ano Lobb, "Hepatoxicity Associated With Weight-Loss Supplements:
    A Case for Better Post-Marketing Surveillance, *World Journal of Gas-
    troenterology* 15, no. 14 (April 14, 2009): 1786–1787, http://www.ncbi
    .nlm.nih.gov/pmc/articles/PMC2668789/ (accessed March 26, 2013).

13. Associated Press, "FDA Warns Consumers to Avoid Brazilian Diet
    Pills," USAToday.com, January 13, 2006, http://usatoday30.usatoday
    .com/news/health/2006-01-13-brazilian-diet-pills_x.htm (accessed
    March 26, 2013).

DON COLBERT, MD, was born in Tupelo, Mississippi. He attended Oral Roberts School of Medicine in Tulsa, Oklahoma, where he received a bachelor of science degree in biology in addition to his degree in medicine. Dr. Colbert completed his internship and residency with Florida Hospital in Orlando, Florida. He is board certified in family practice and anti-aging medicine and has received extensive training in nutritional medicine.

If you would like more information about natural and divine healing, or information about *Divine Health nutritional products*, you may contact Dr. Colbert at:

Don Colbert, MD
1908 Boothe Circle
Longwood, FL 32750
Telephone: 407-331-7007 (for ordering products only)
Website: www.drcolbert.com.

Disclaimer: Dr. Colbert and the staff of Divine Health Wellness Center are prohibited from addressing a patient's medical condition by phone, facsimile, or e-mail. Please refer questions related to your medical condition to your own primary care physician.

Pick up these other great Bible Cure books by Don Colbert, MD: